THIS BOOK BELONGS TO
A WONDERFUL SOUL
NAMED:

A DEDICATION
FOR
YSA

Dearest YSA,

Those of us who are lucky enough to know you can attest to your resilience when facing life's challenges. First, this book is dedicated to you. I wrote this, to honor your light and your quiet strength to continue shining brightly even in the darkest times. As you share your story, may your vulnerability and perseverance foster connection, comfort, and hope for others on a similar journey. With each passing year and every milestone, the person you are becoming reflects your generous heart and loving spirit. May your recent victories continue to cultivate deep gratitude within you, spreading joy, love, and encouragement to all those whose lives you touch. To witness your journey has been nothing less than inspirational. I am in awe of you, my friend. And so, my spirit would also spread this love to everyone who has longed for parenthood while bravely enduring the heartaches along the way. If you've ever questioned your body and mind, shed countless tears, and whispered fervent prayers for your desire to start a family, this book is from my heart to yours.

Always grateful,

CHRISTINA

This book serves as a touching love
letter from a couple yearning to
become parents. It is penned from a
mother's perspective who, after a
lengthy wait, finally experiences the
gentle flutter of new life growing inside
her. Through lyrical verses and
whimsical illustrations, this tale
celebrates both the challenges and
joys of the pregnancy journey, as well
as the deep connection between a
mother and her child.

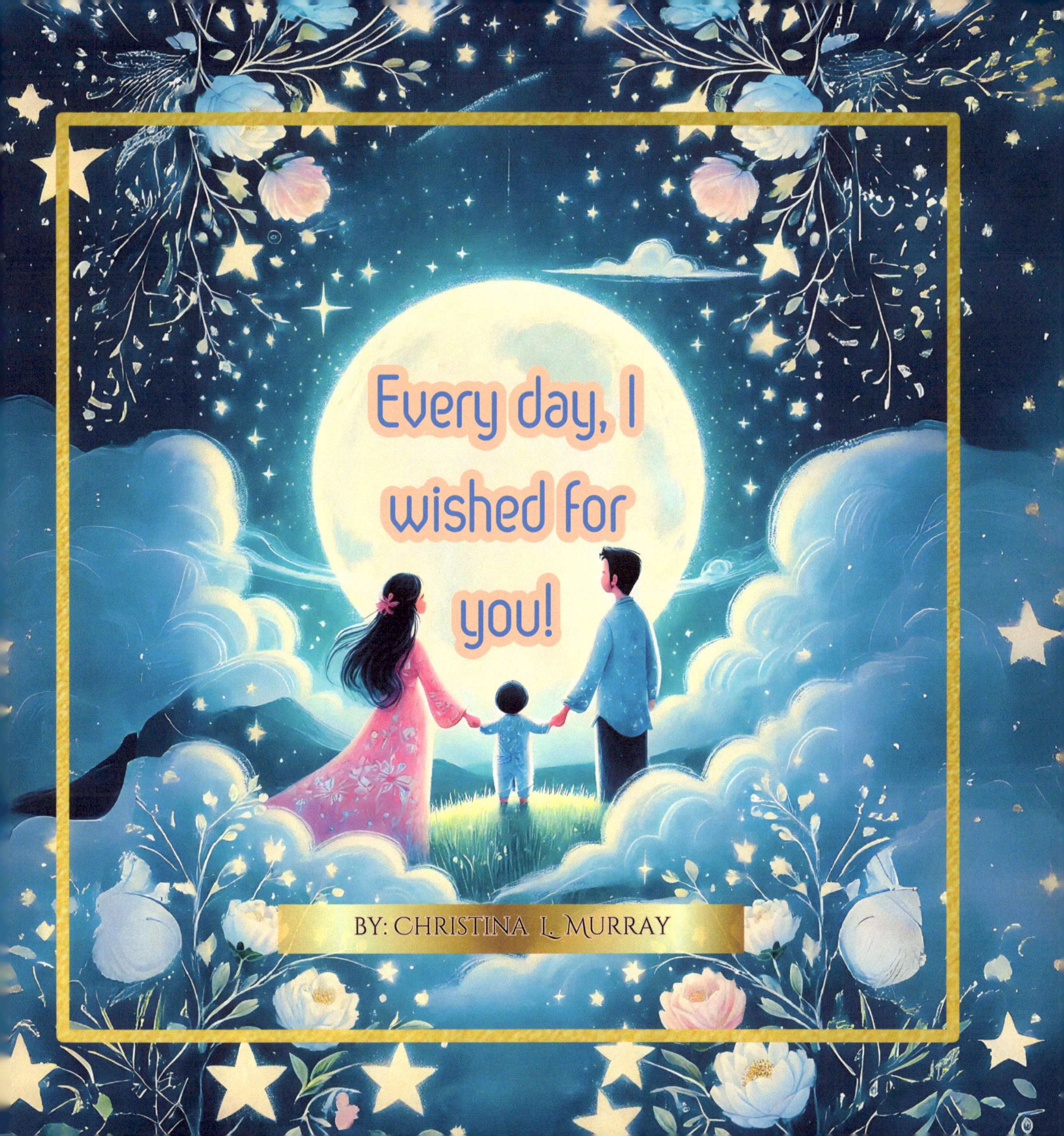

Every day, I wished for you!
BY: CHRISTINA L. MURRAY

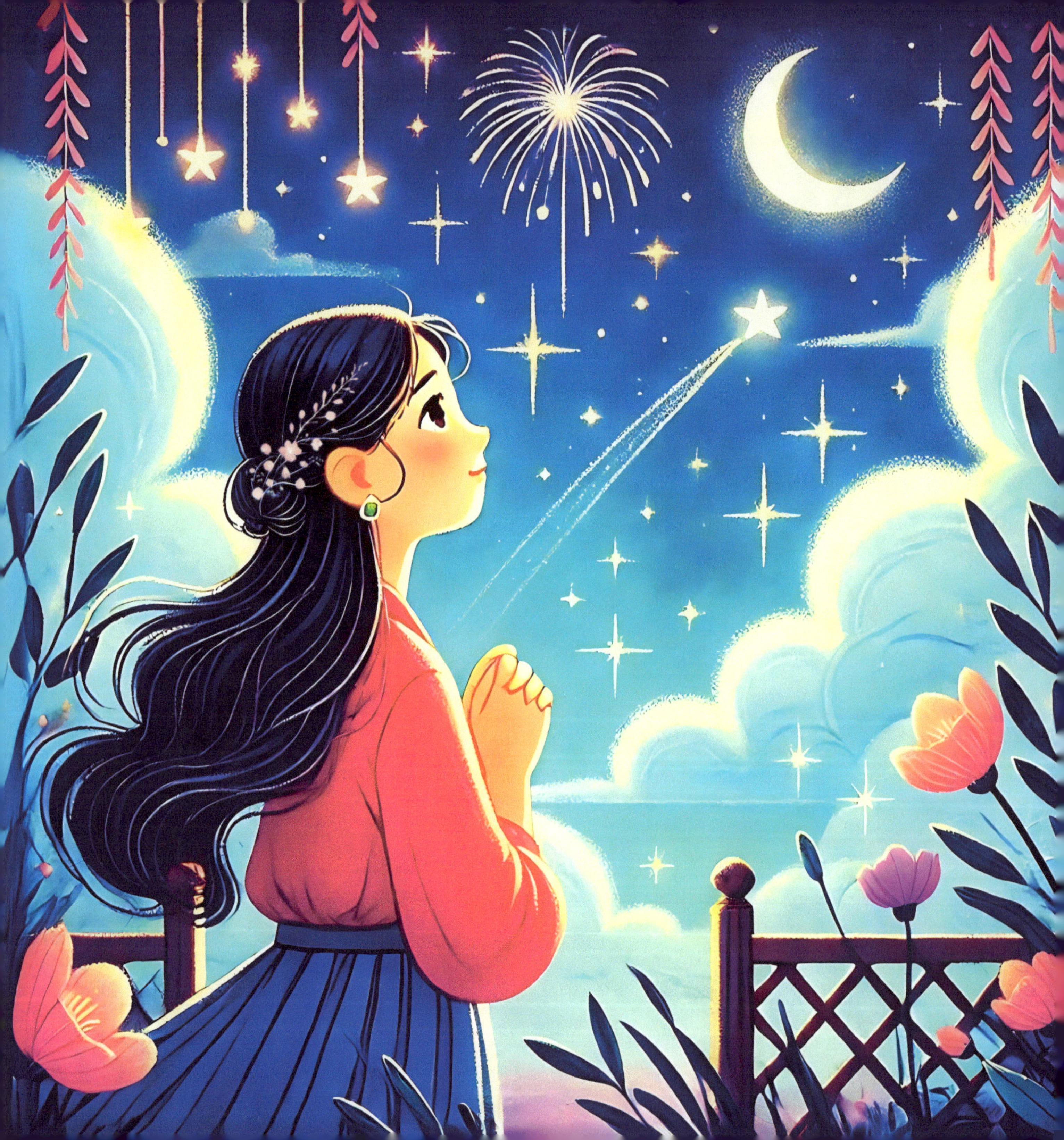

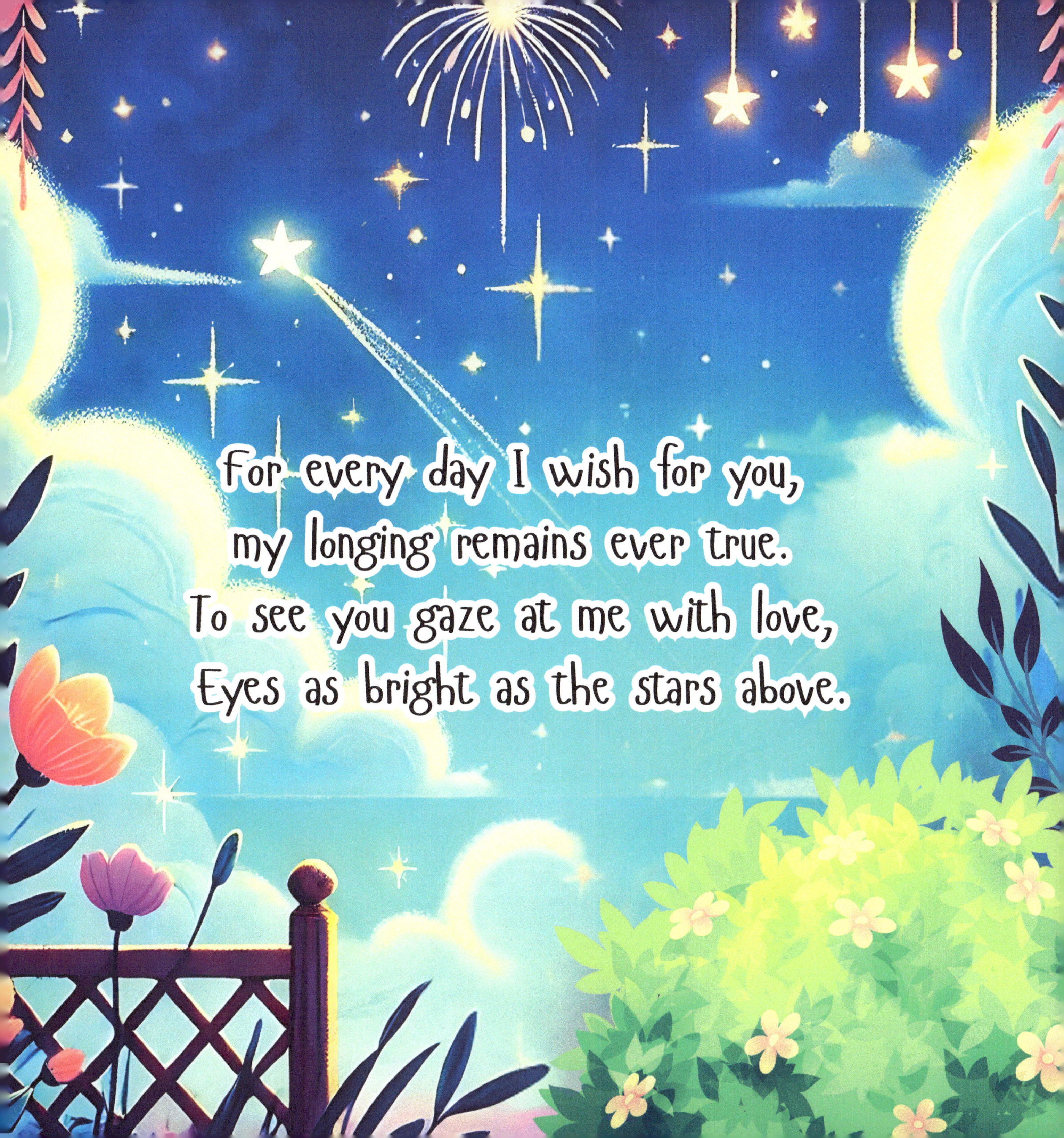

For every day I wish for you,
my longing remains ever true.
To see you gaze at me with love,
Eyes as bright as the stars above.

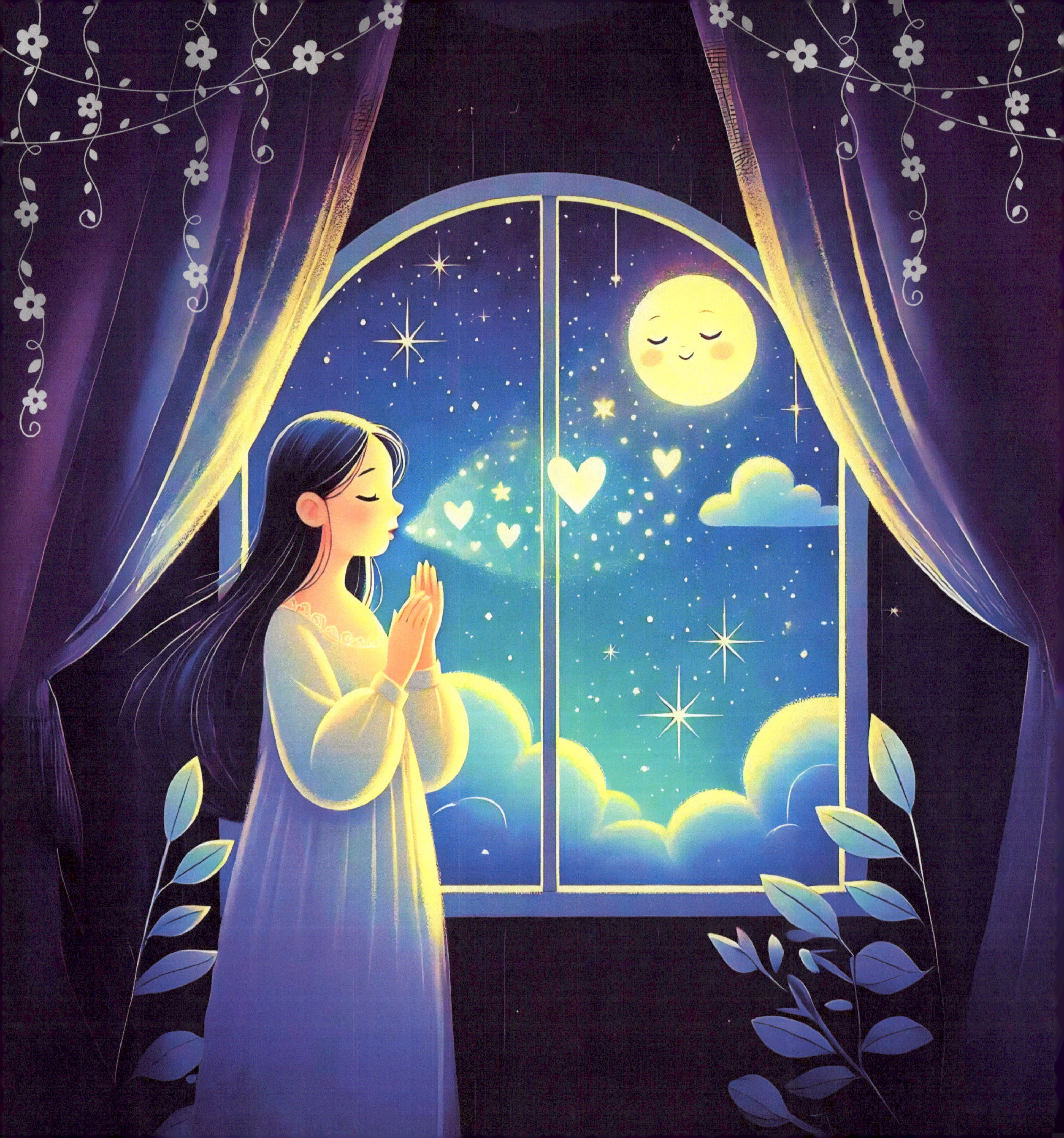

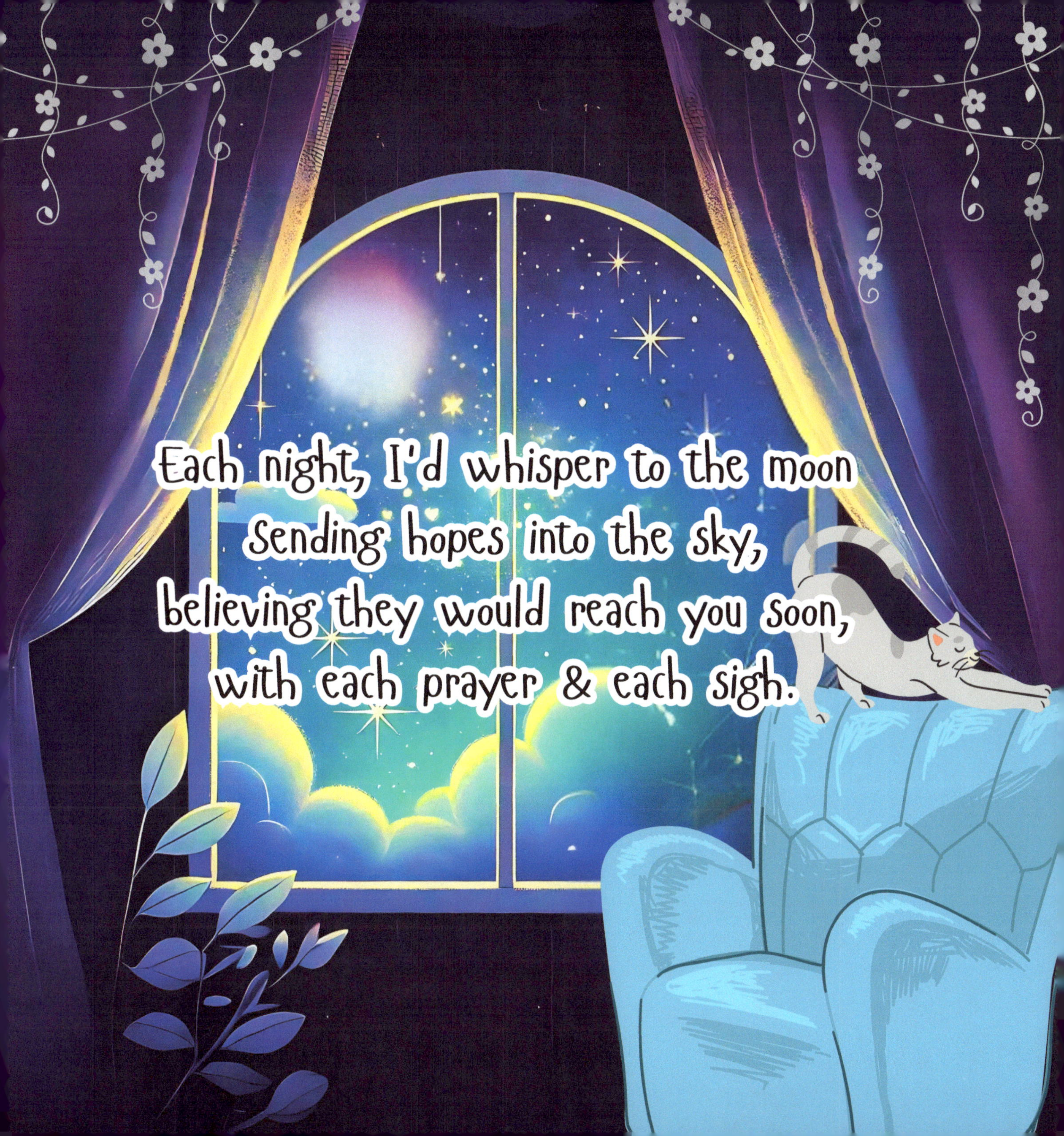

Each night, I'd whisper to the moon
Sending hopes into the sky,
believing they would reach you soon,
with each prayer & each sigh.

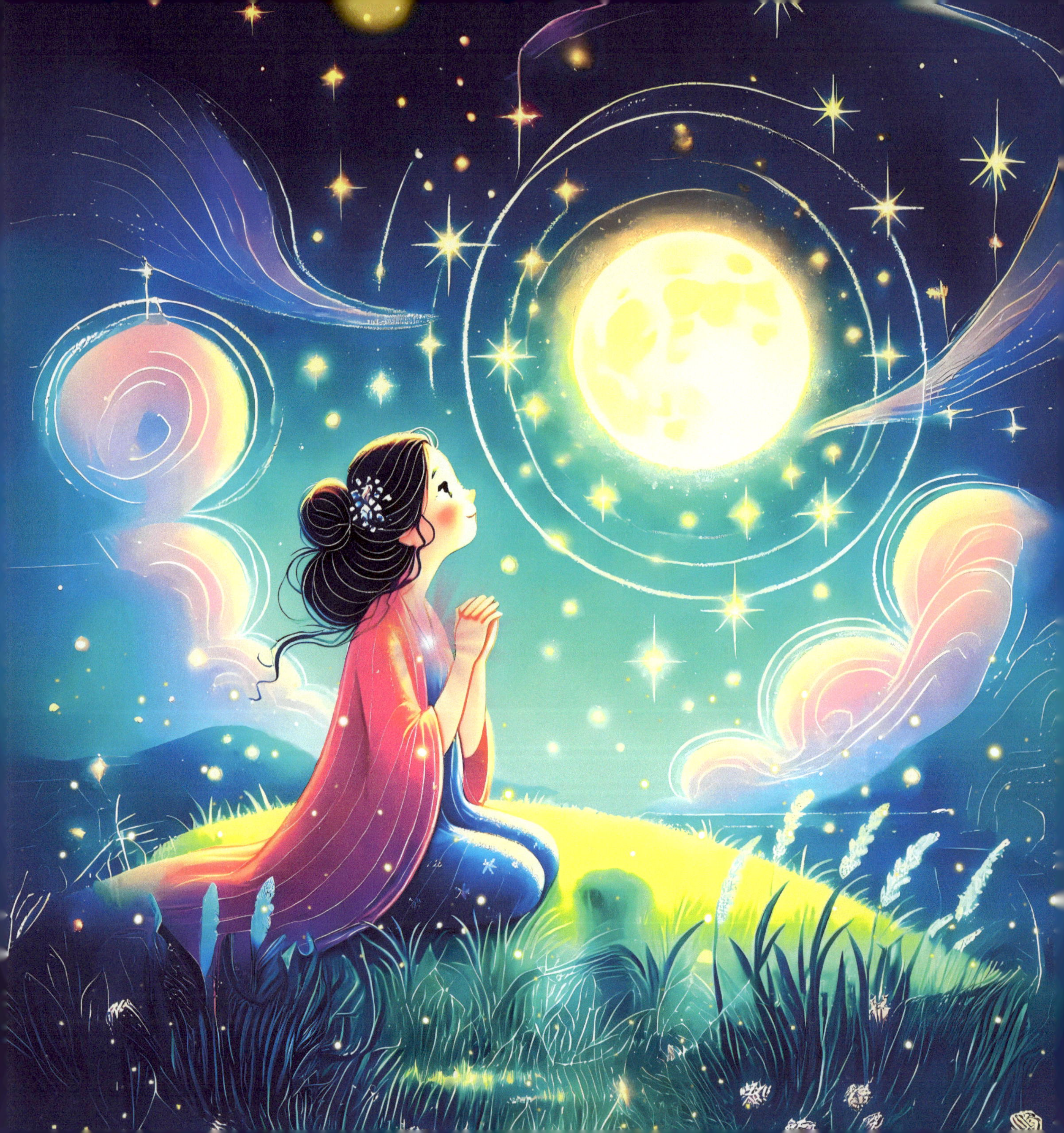

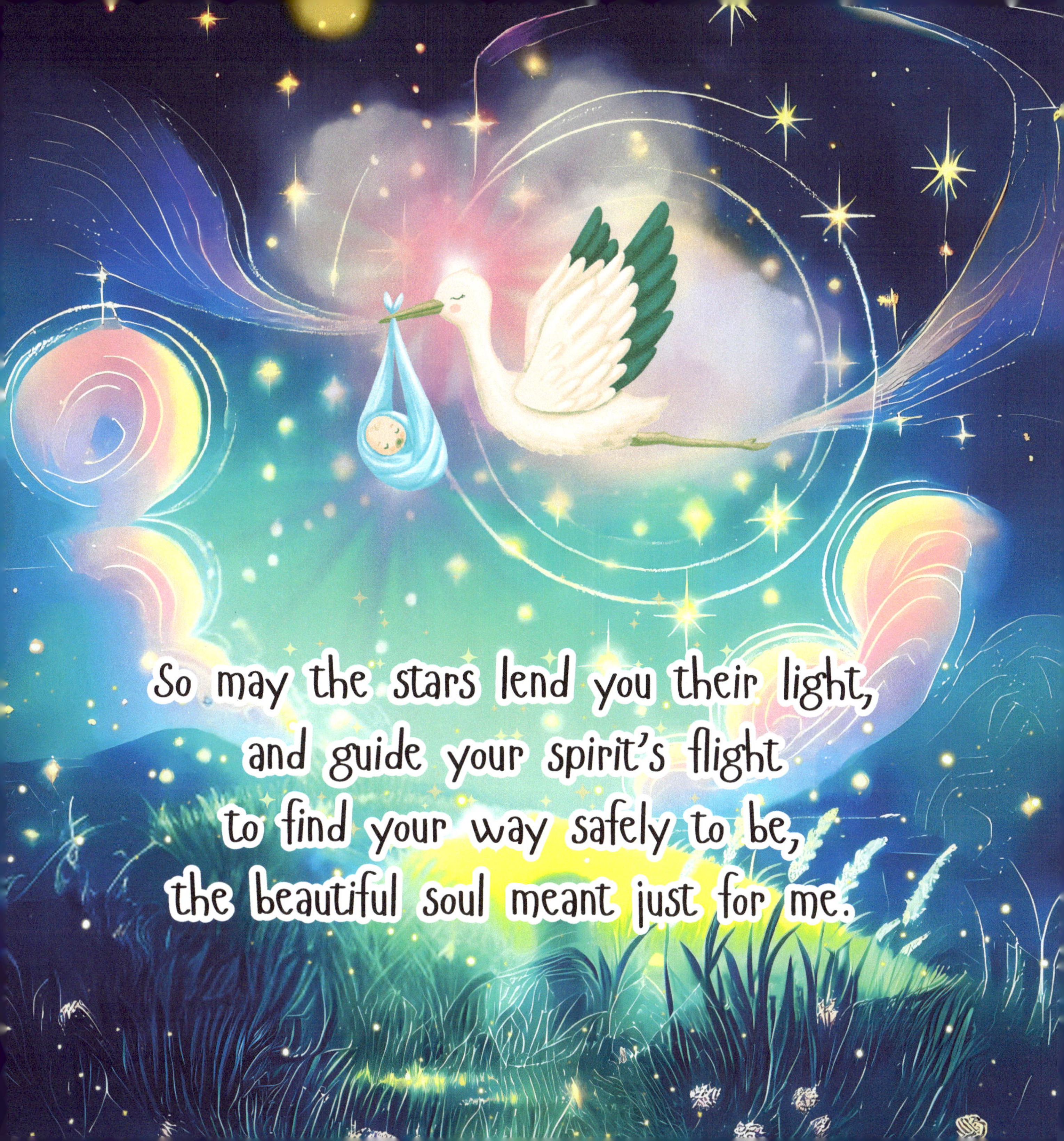
So may the stars lend you their light,
and guide your spirit's flight
to find your way safely to be,
the beautiful soul meant just for me.

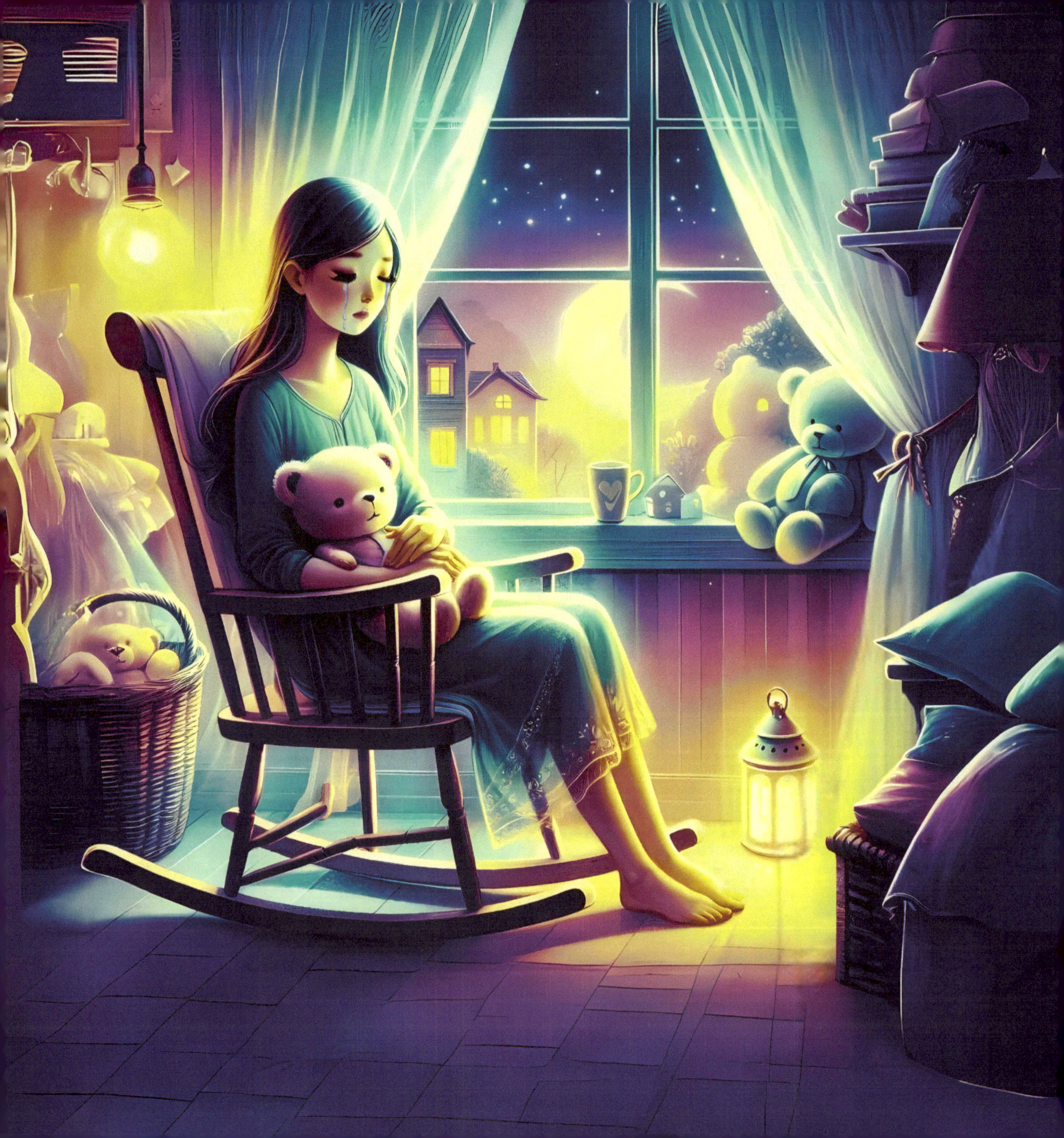

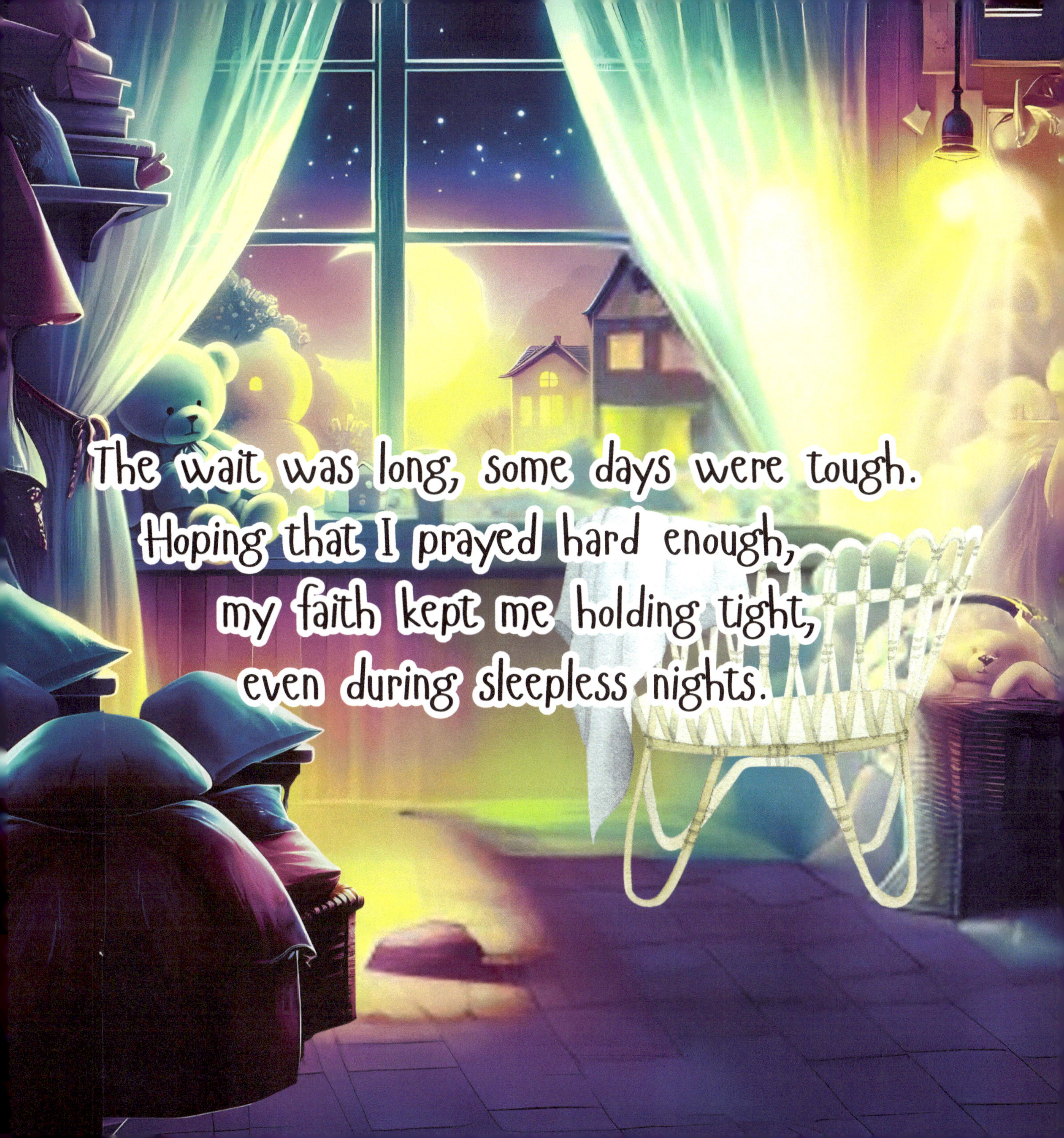
The wait was long, some days were tough.
Hoping that I prayed hard enough,
my faith kept me holding tight,
even during sleepless nights.

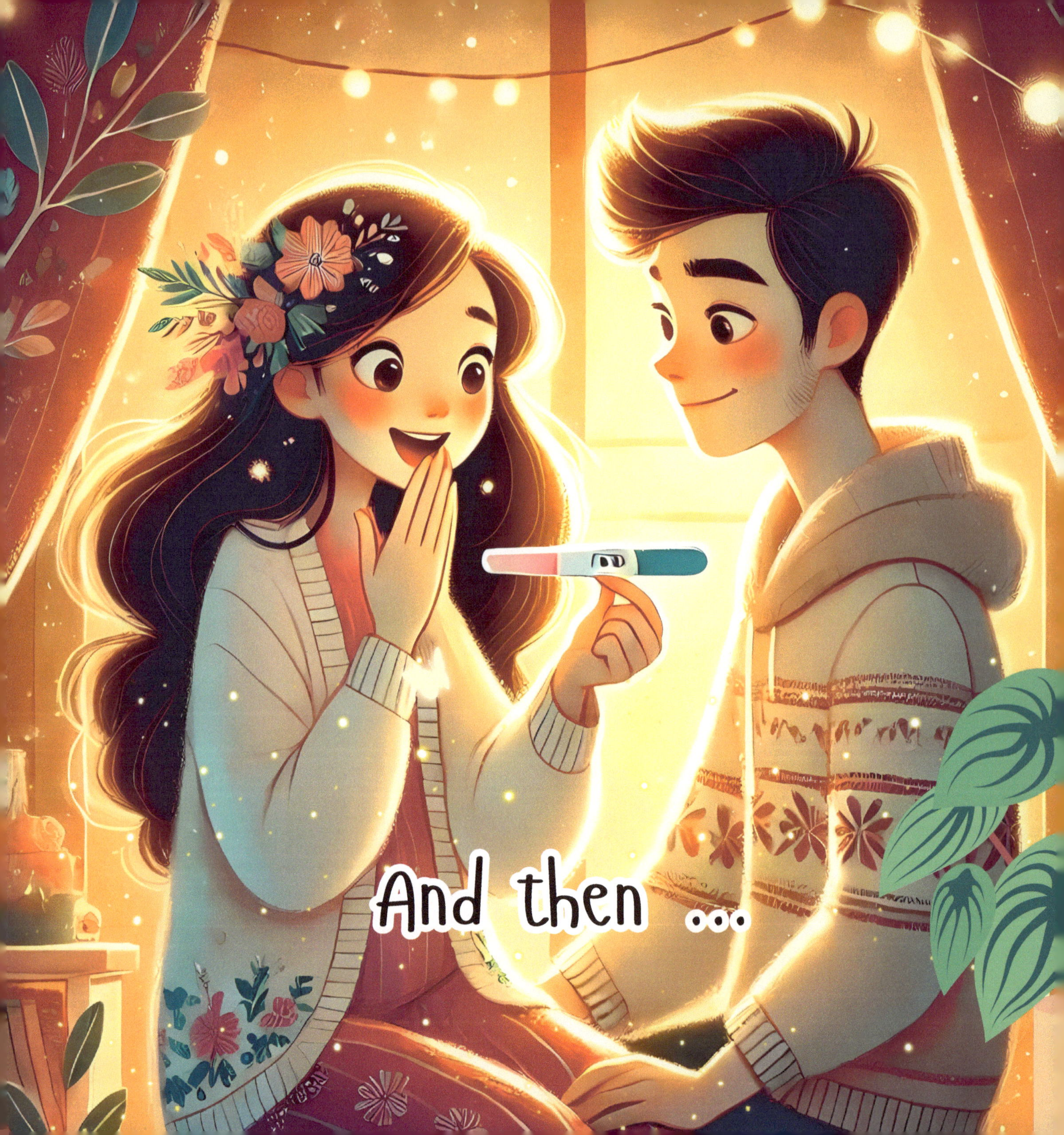
And then ...

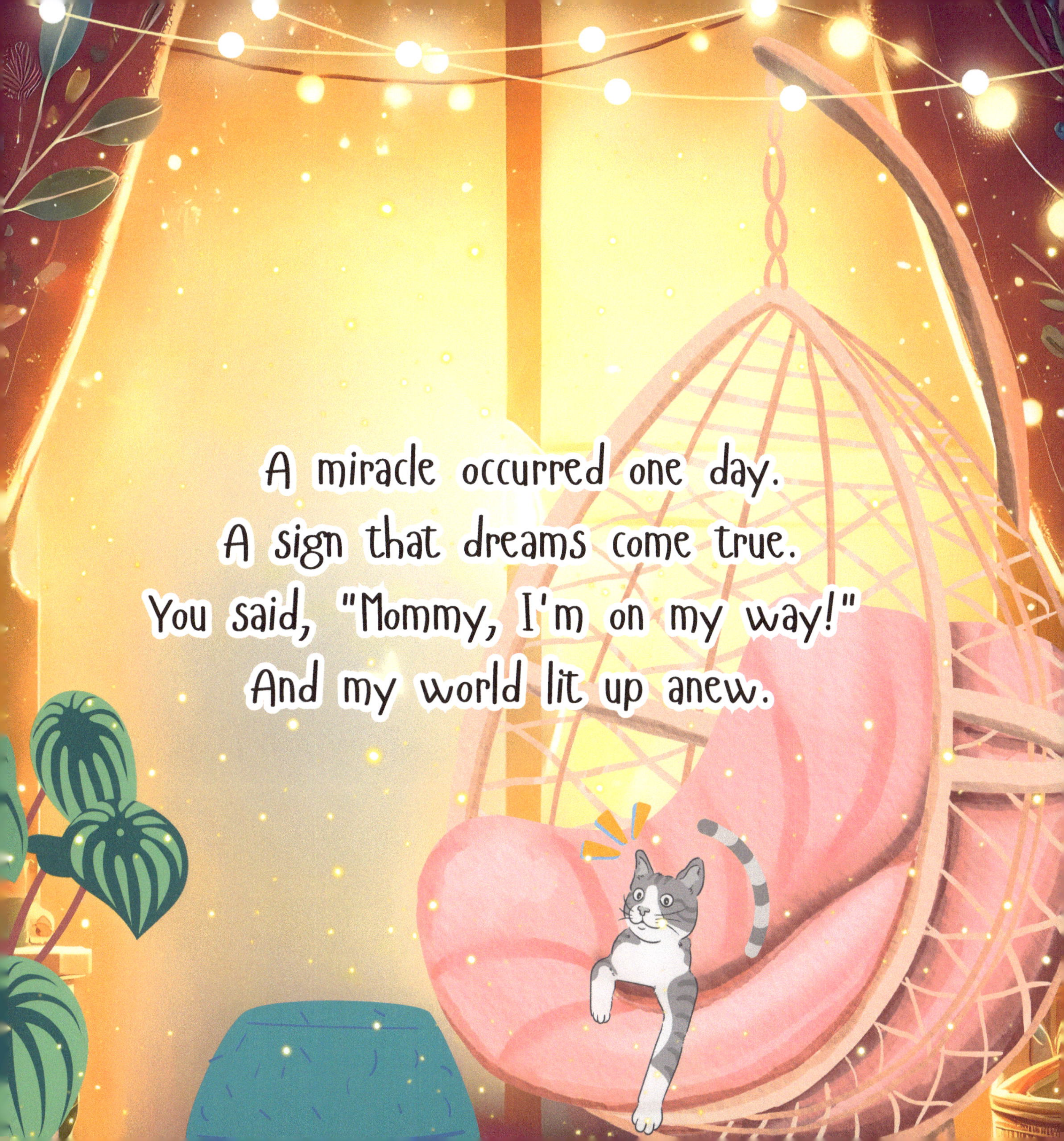

A miracle occurred one day.
A sign that dreams come true.
You said, "Mommy, I'm on my way!"
And my world lit up anew.

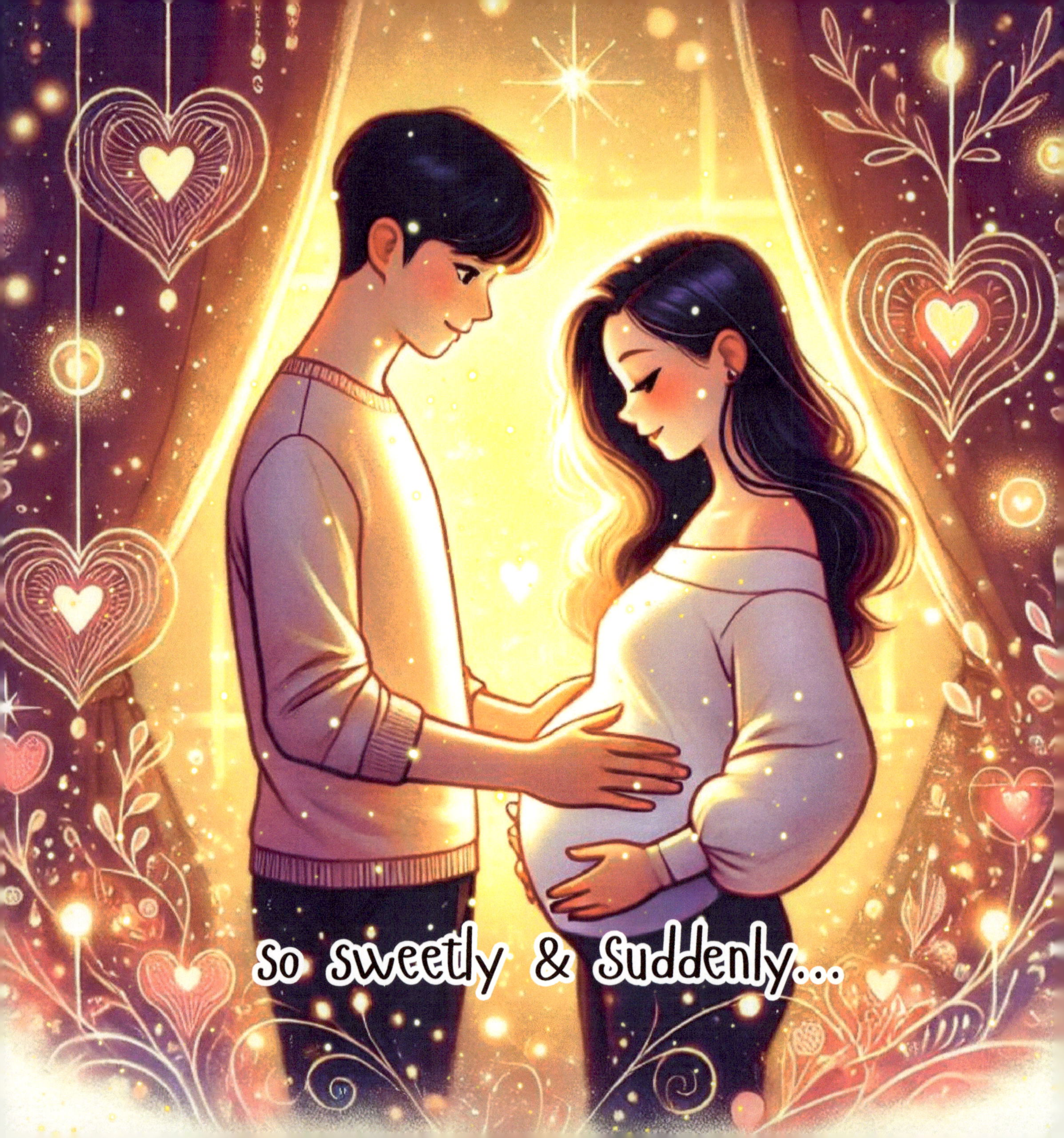
so sweetly & suddenly...

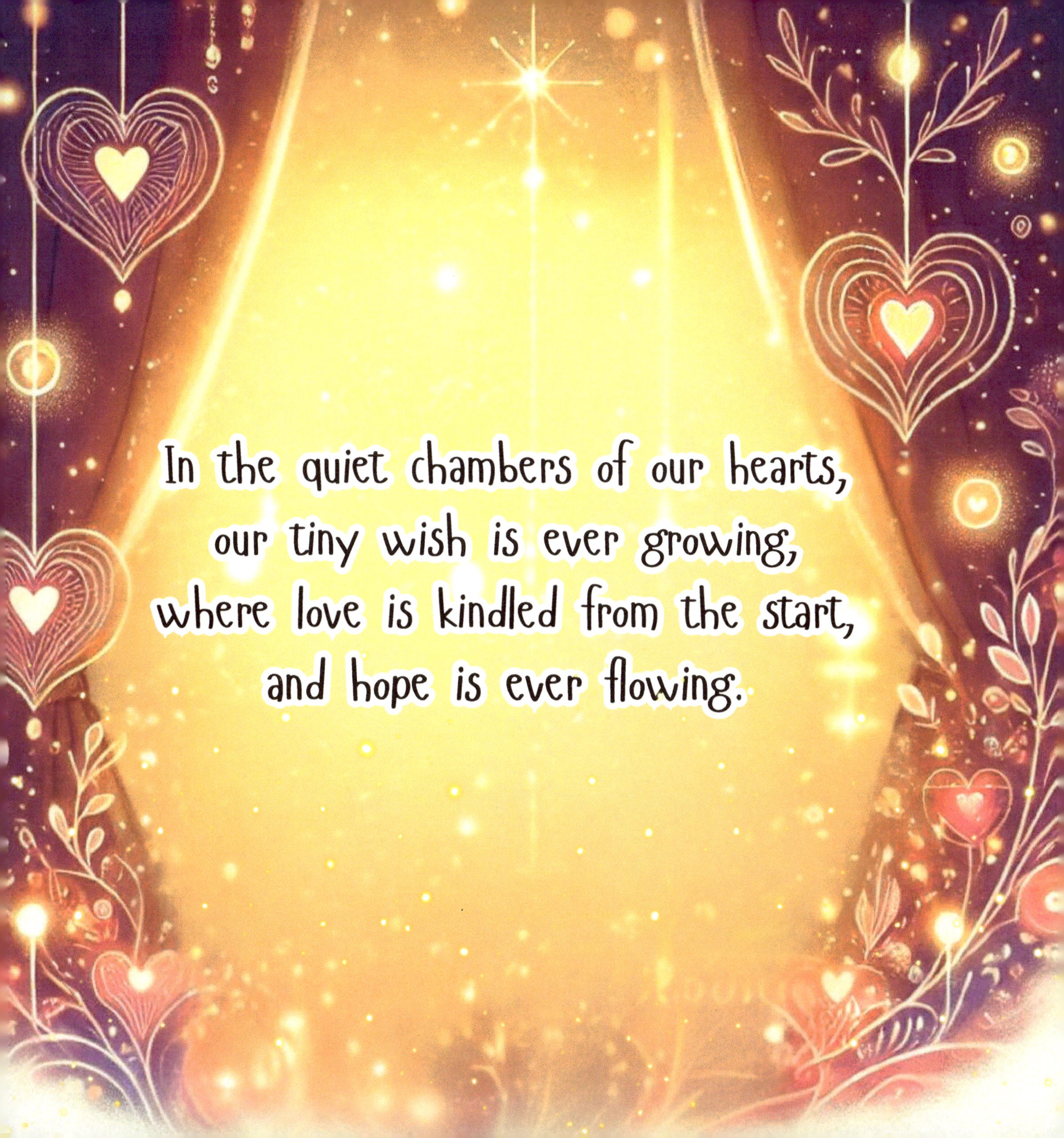

In the quiet chambers of our hearts,
our tiny wish is ever growing,
where love is kindled from the start,
and hope is ever flowing.

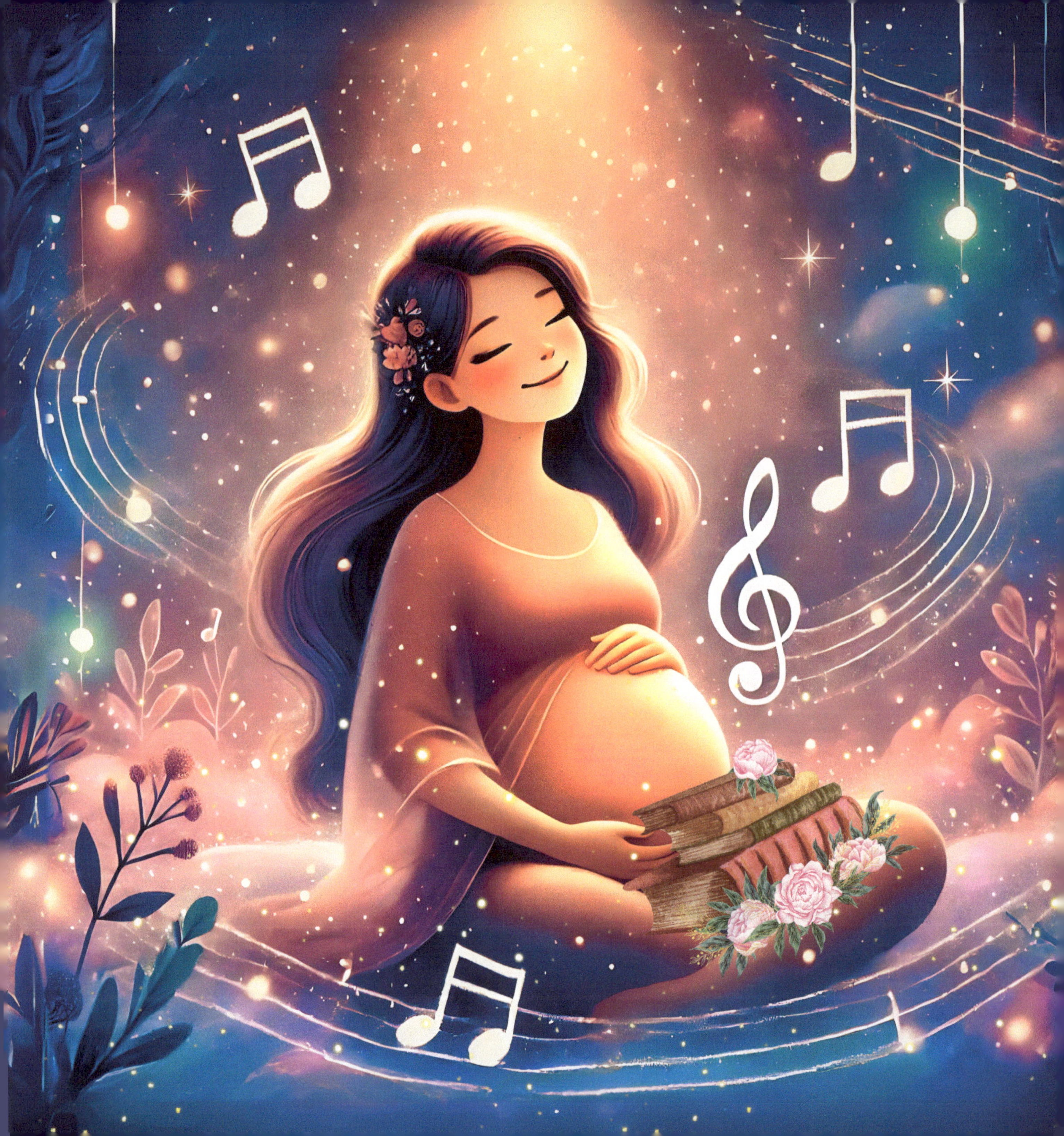

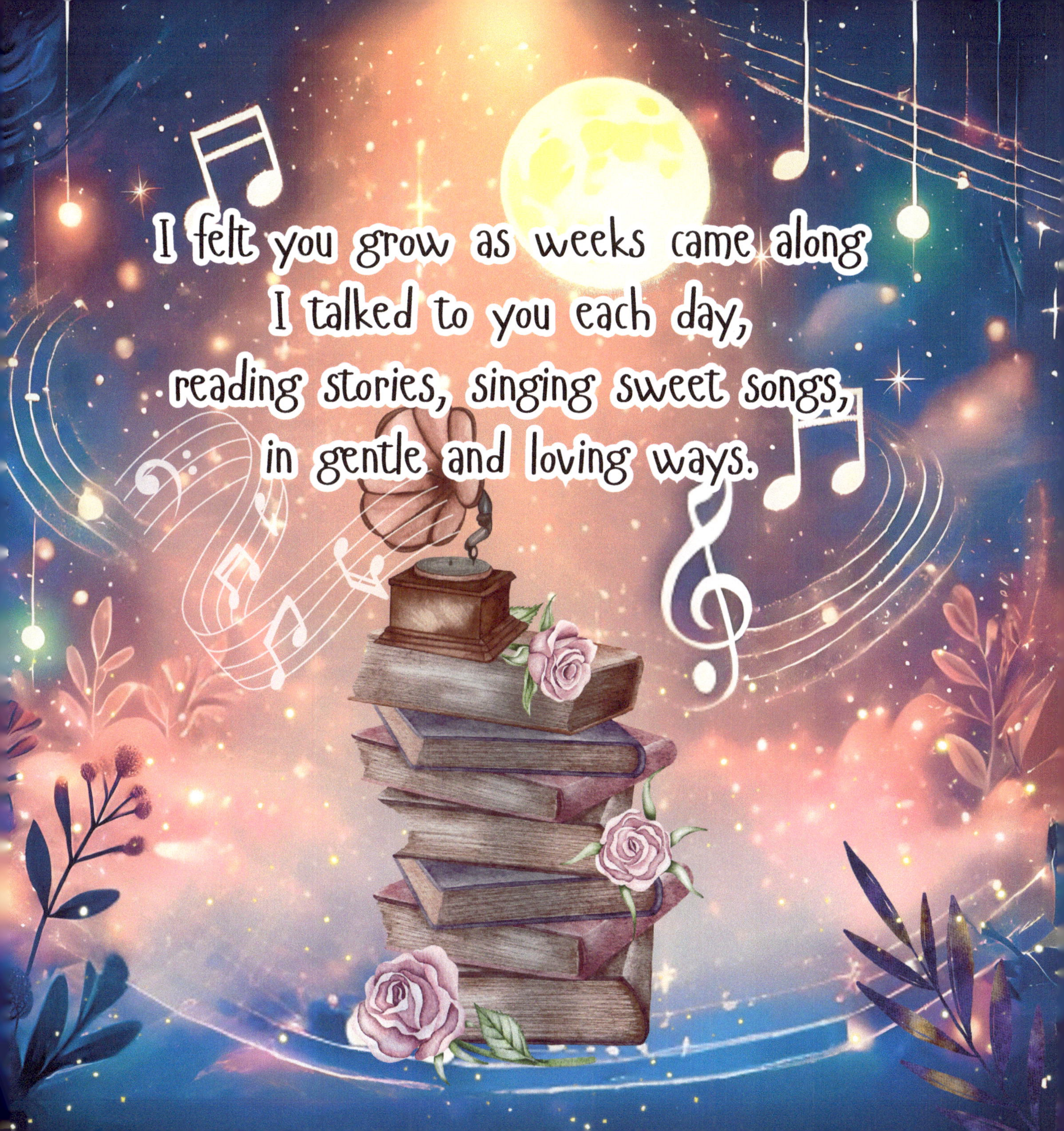

I felt you grow as weeks came along
I talked to you each day,
reading stories, singing sweet songs,
in gentle and loving ways.

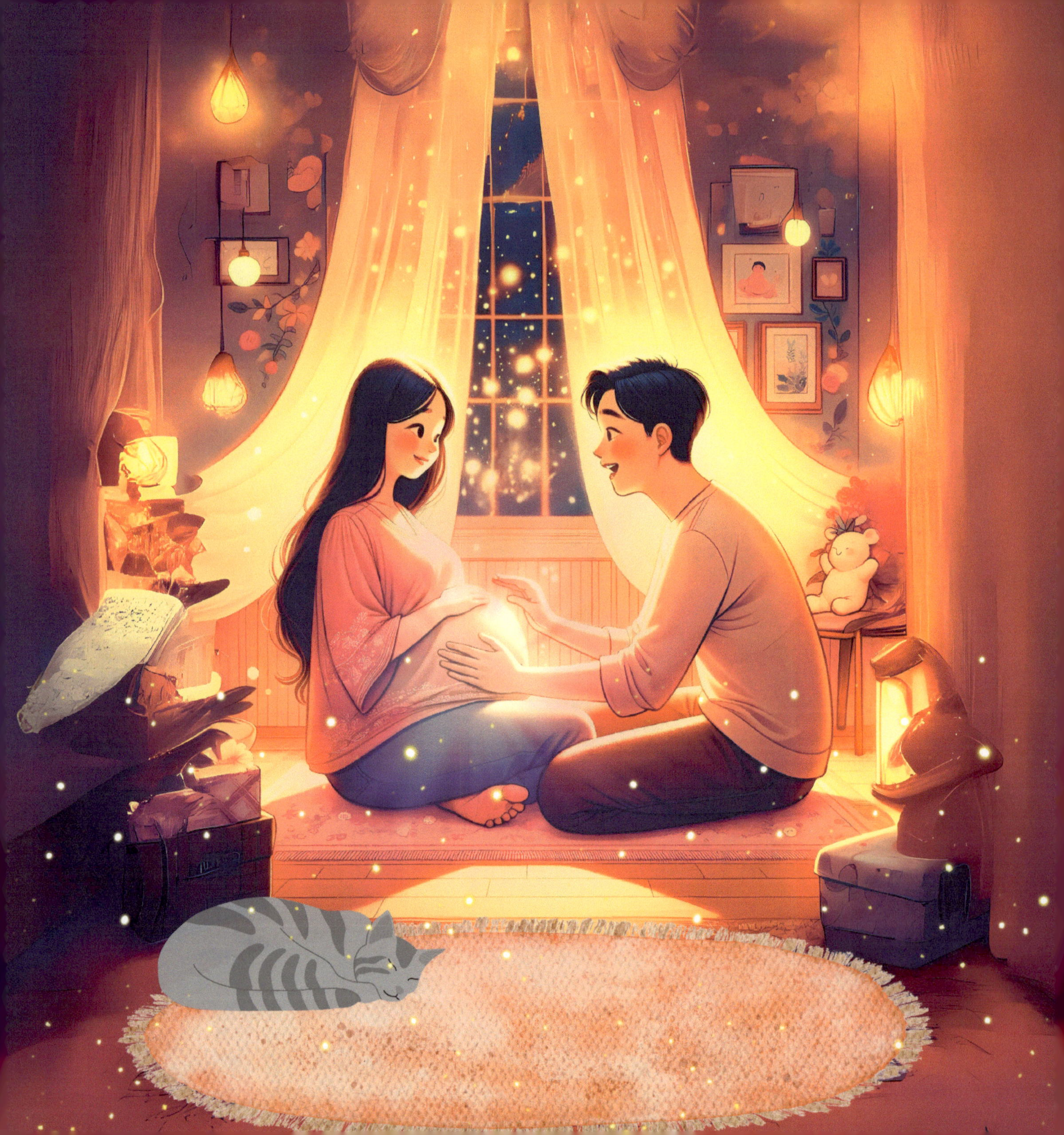

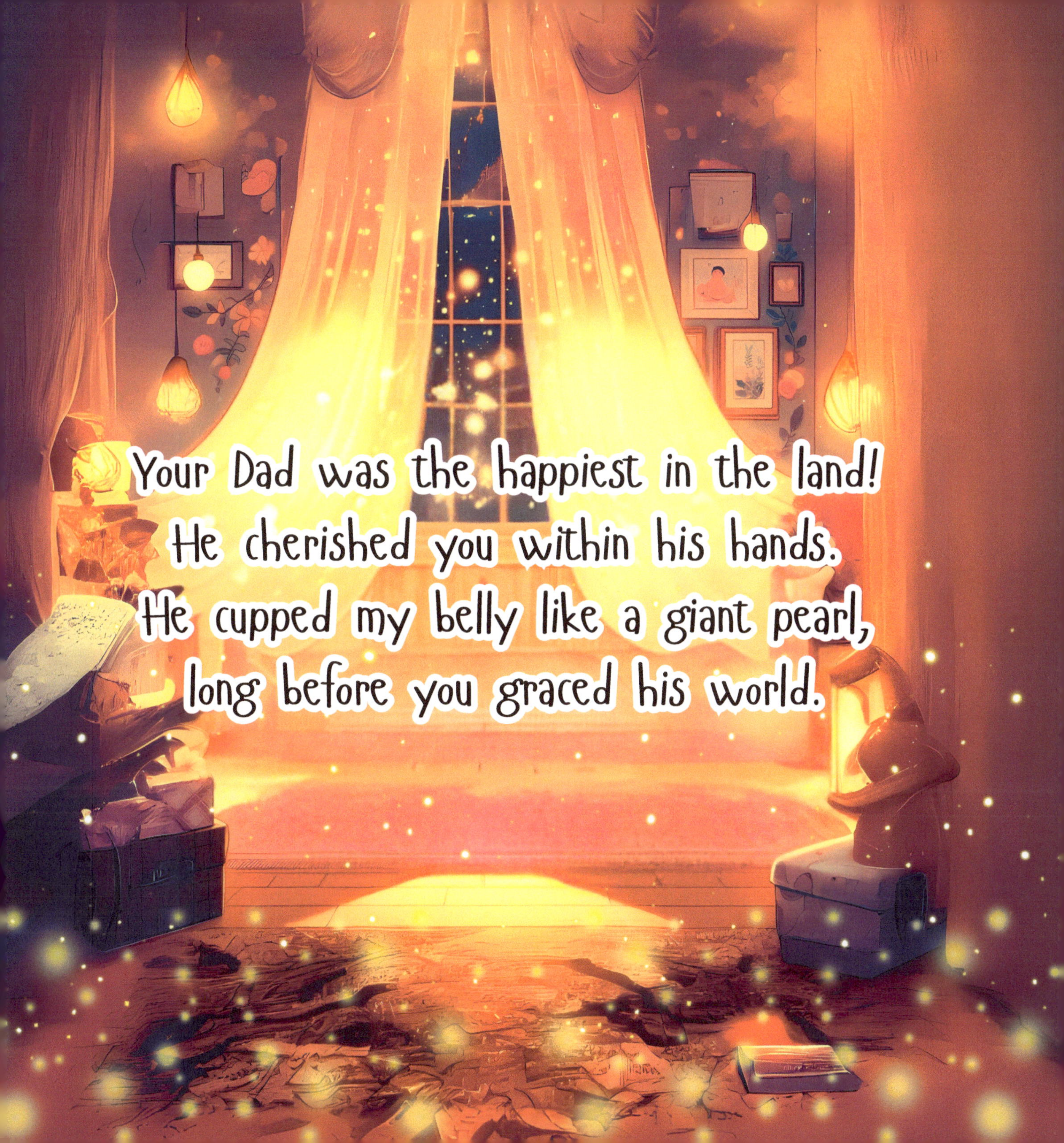

Your Dad was the happiest in the land!
He cherished you within his hands.
He cupped my belly like a giant pearl,
long before you graced his world.

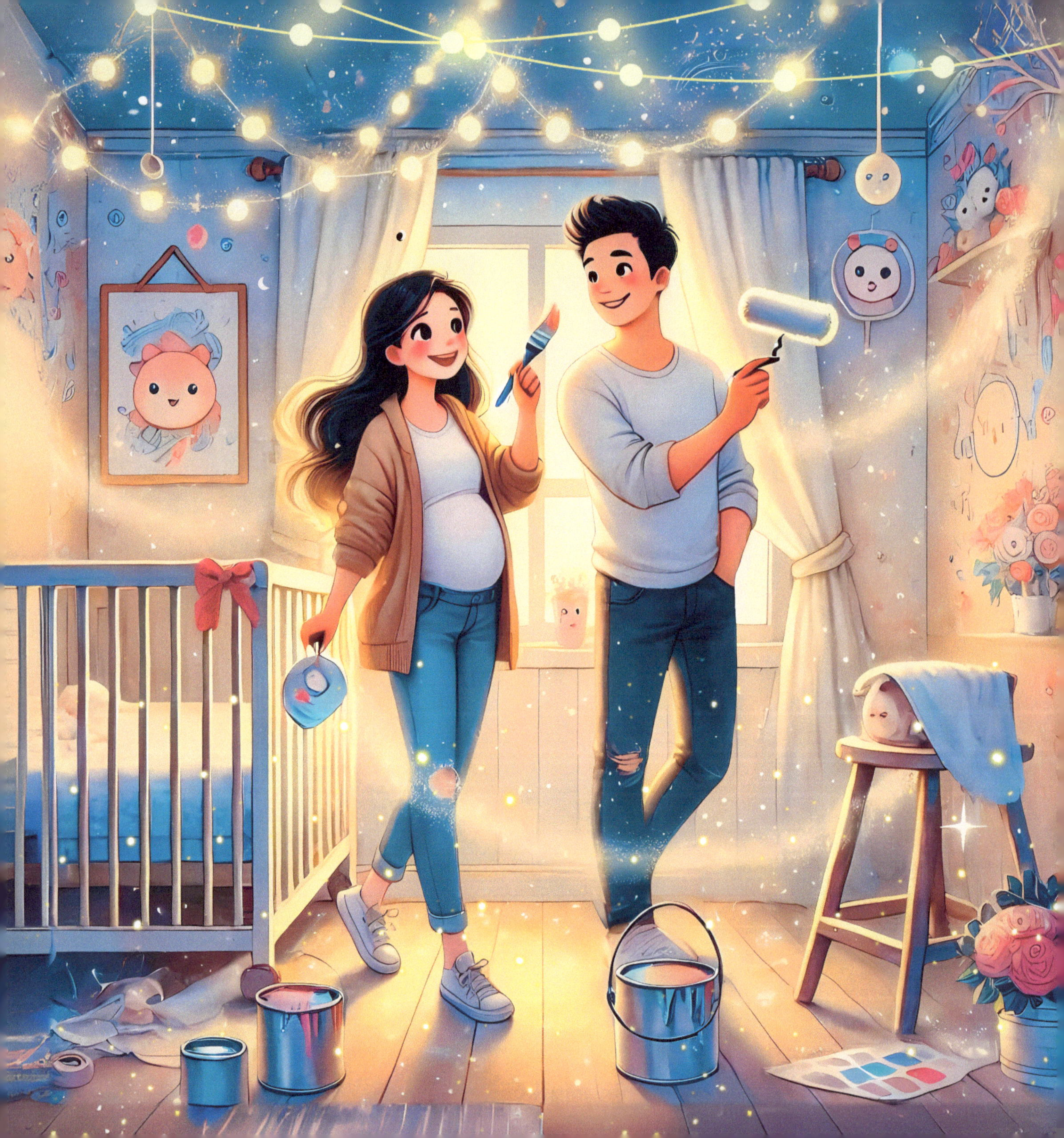

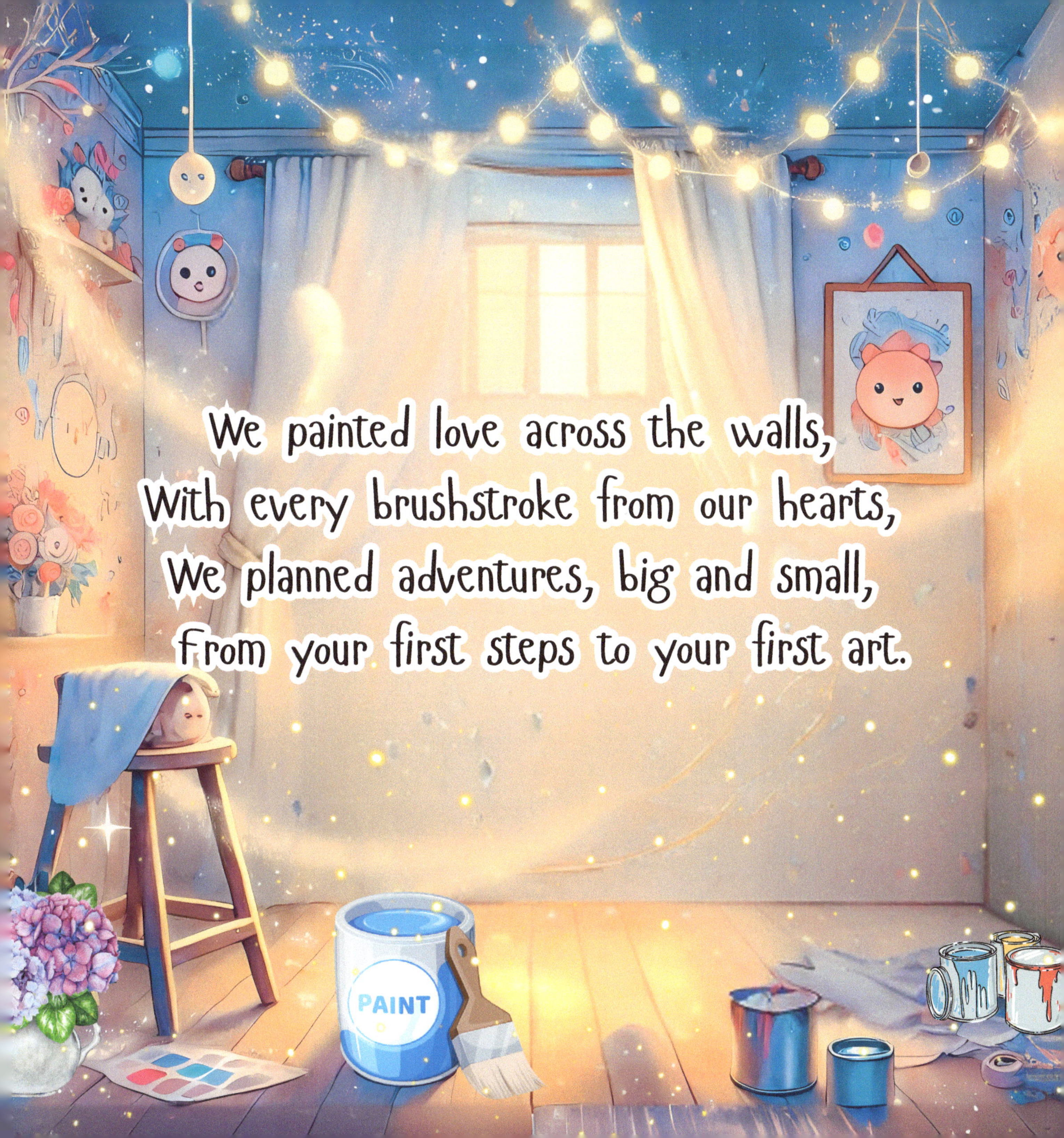
We painted love across the walls,
With every brushstroke from our hearts,
We planned adventures, big and small,
From your first steps to your first art.

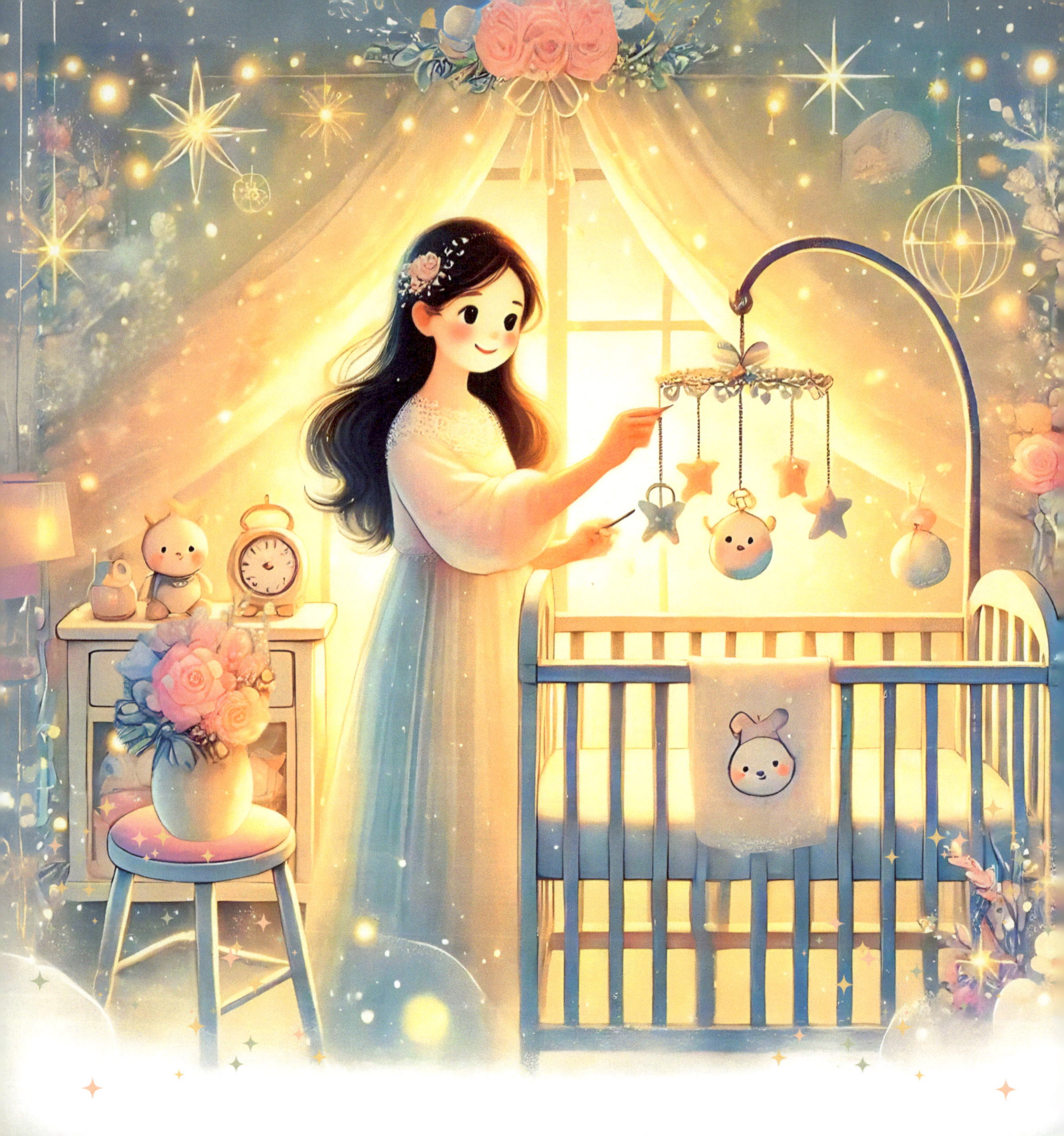

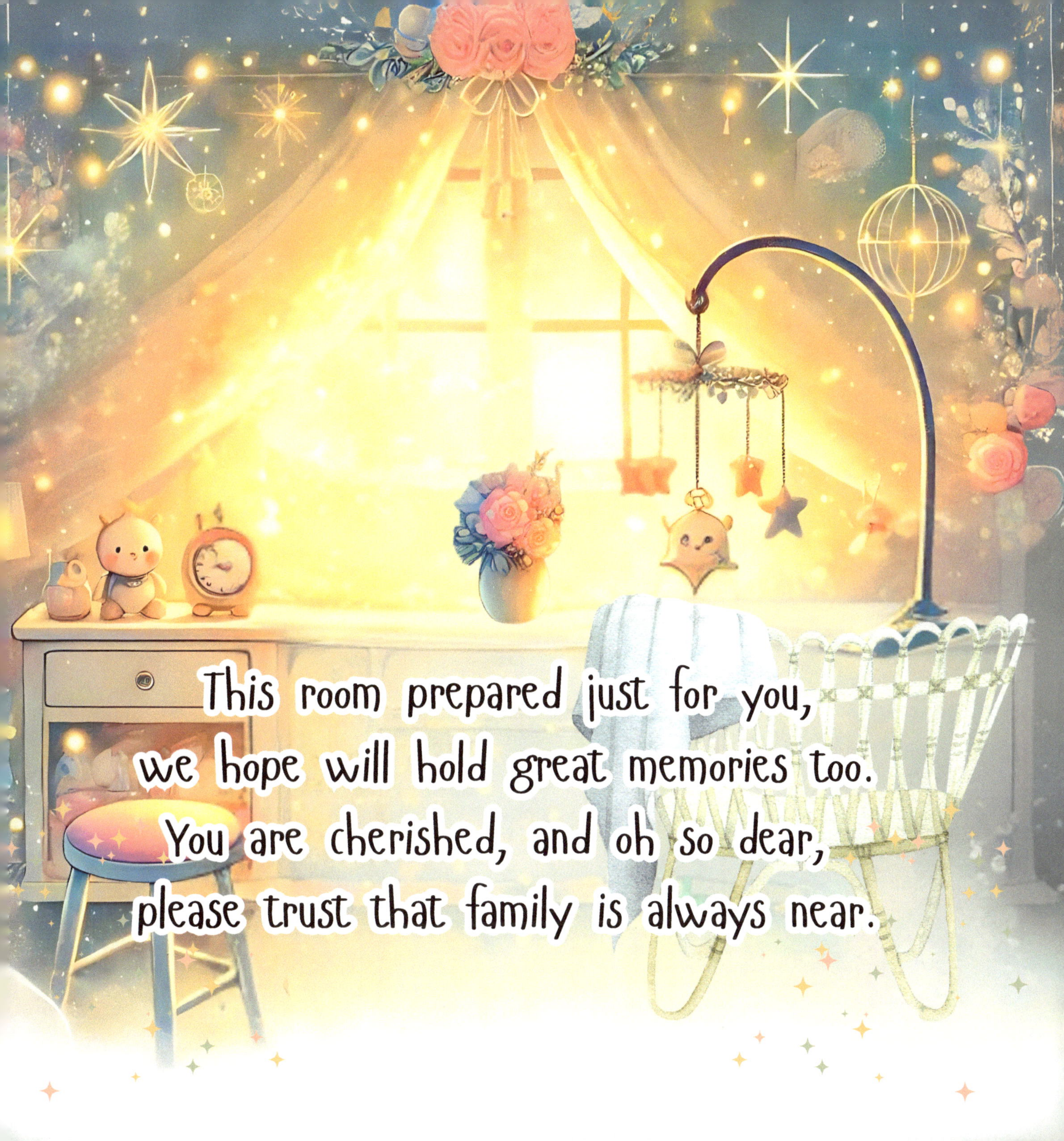
This room prepared just for you,
we hope will hold great memories too.
You are cherished, and oh so dear,
please trust that family is always near.

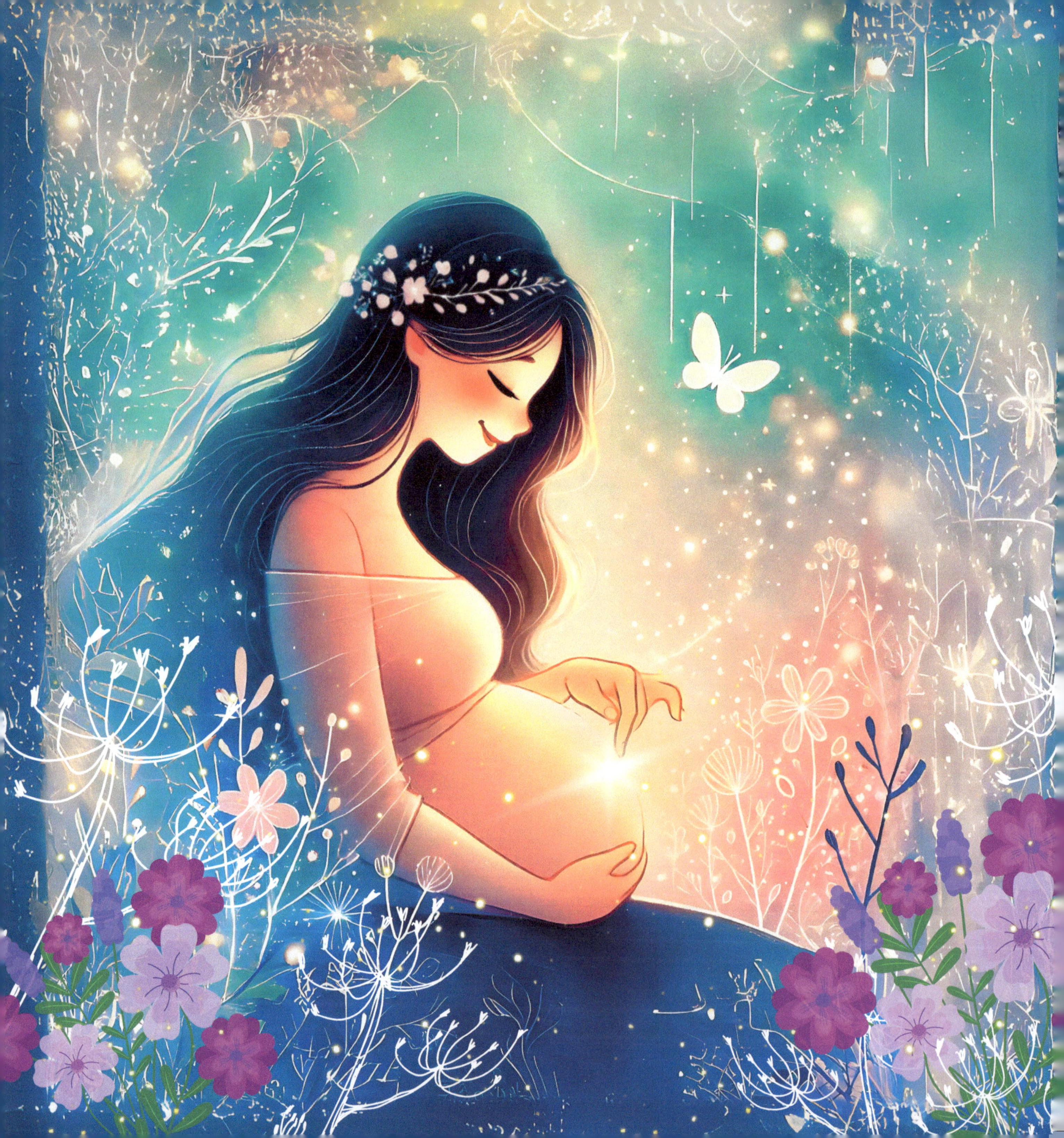

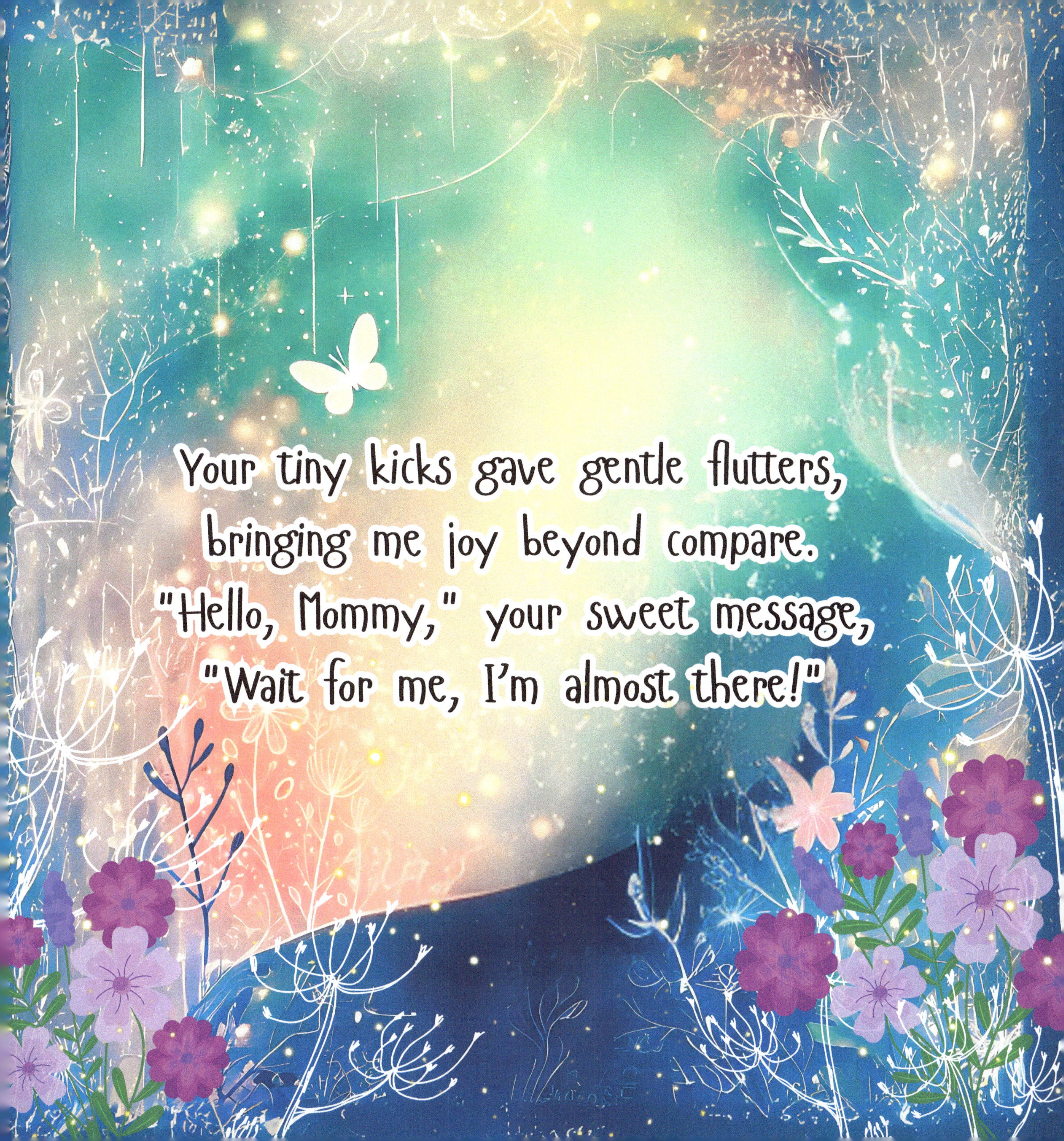
Your tiny kicks gave gentle flutters,
bringing me joy beyond compare.
"Hello, Mommy," your sweet message,
"Wait for me, I'm almost there!"

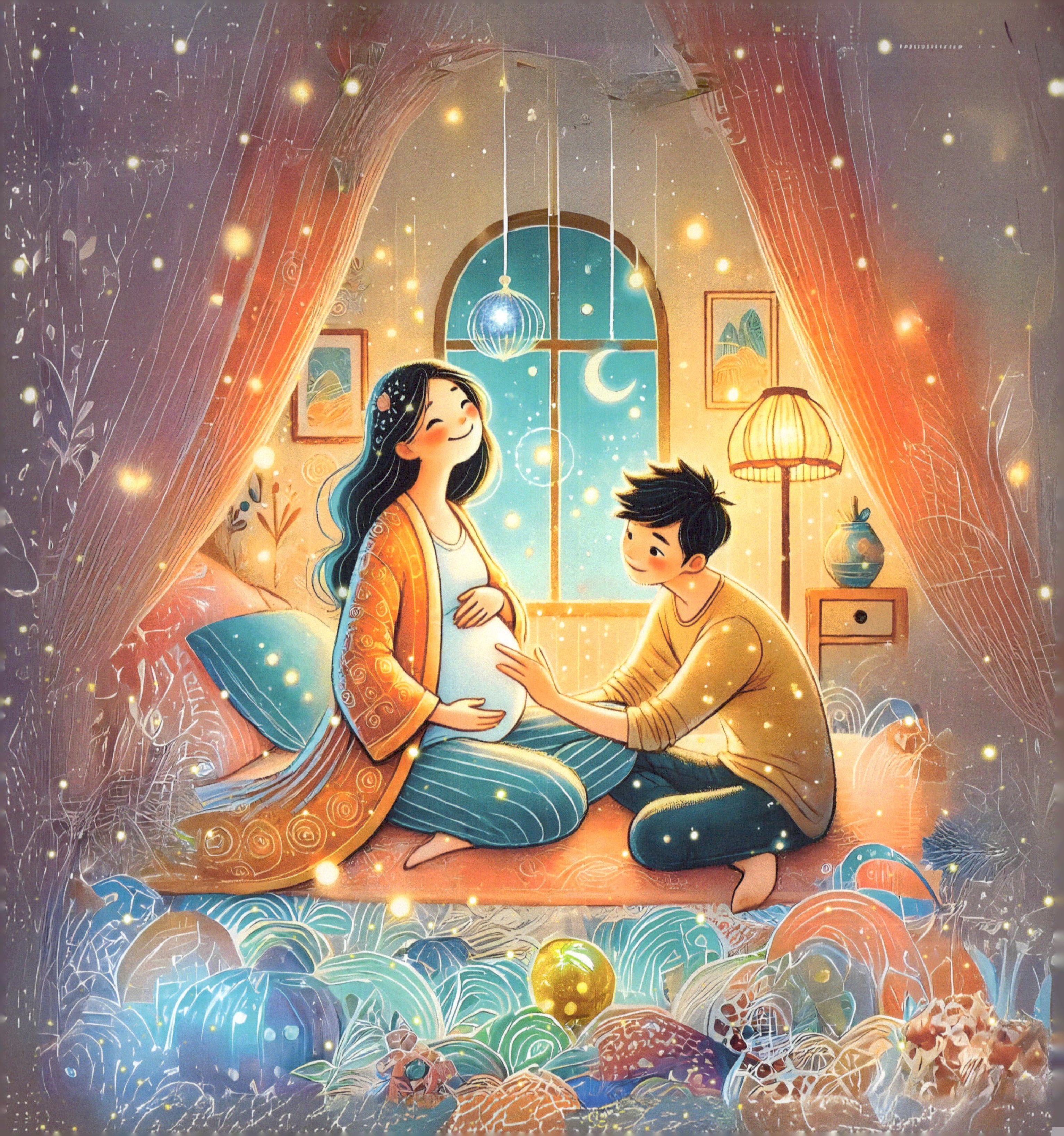

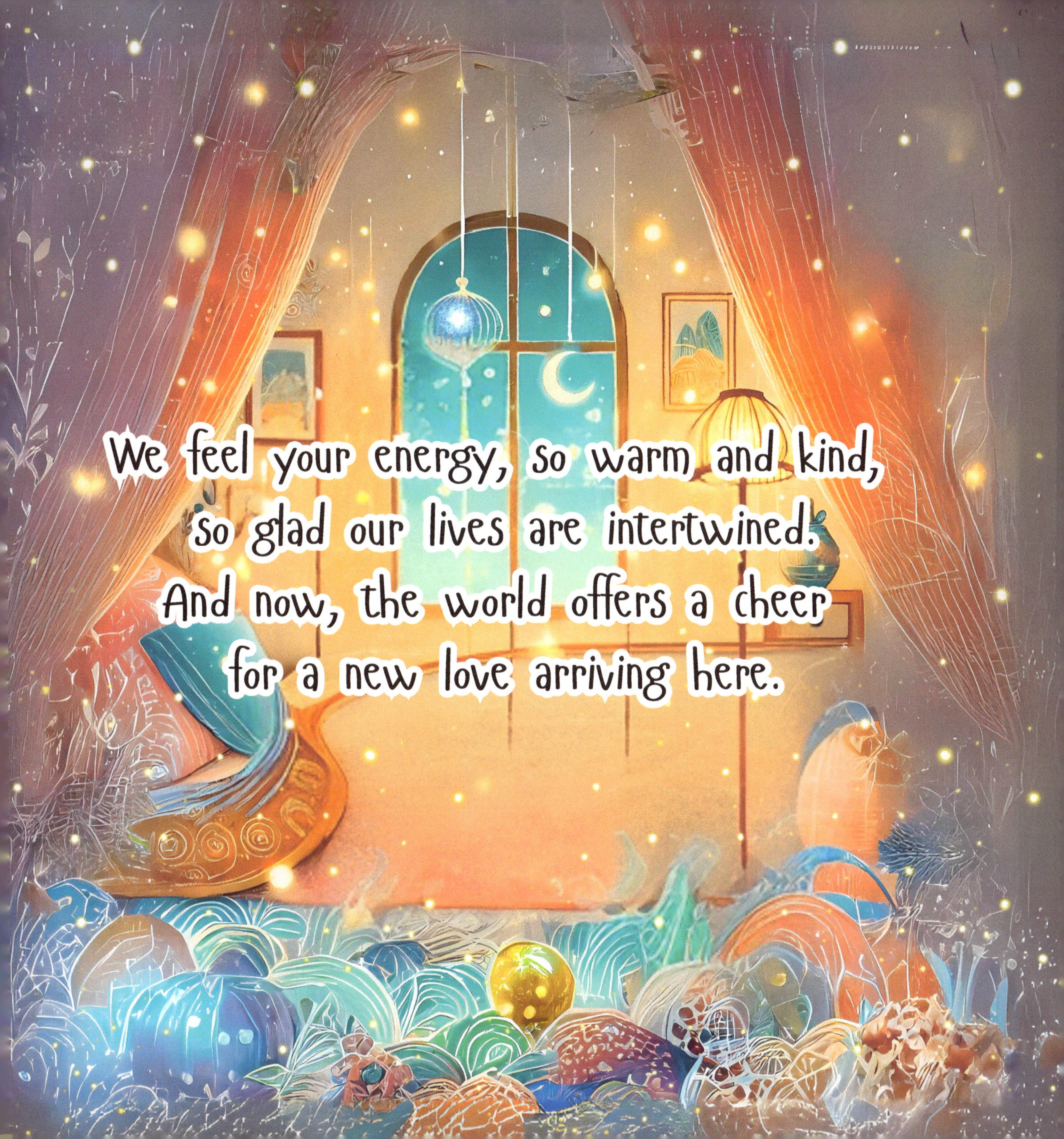

We feel your energy, so warm and kind,
so glad our lives are intertwined.
And now, the world offers a cheer
for a new love arriving here.

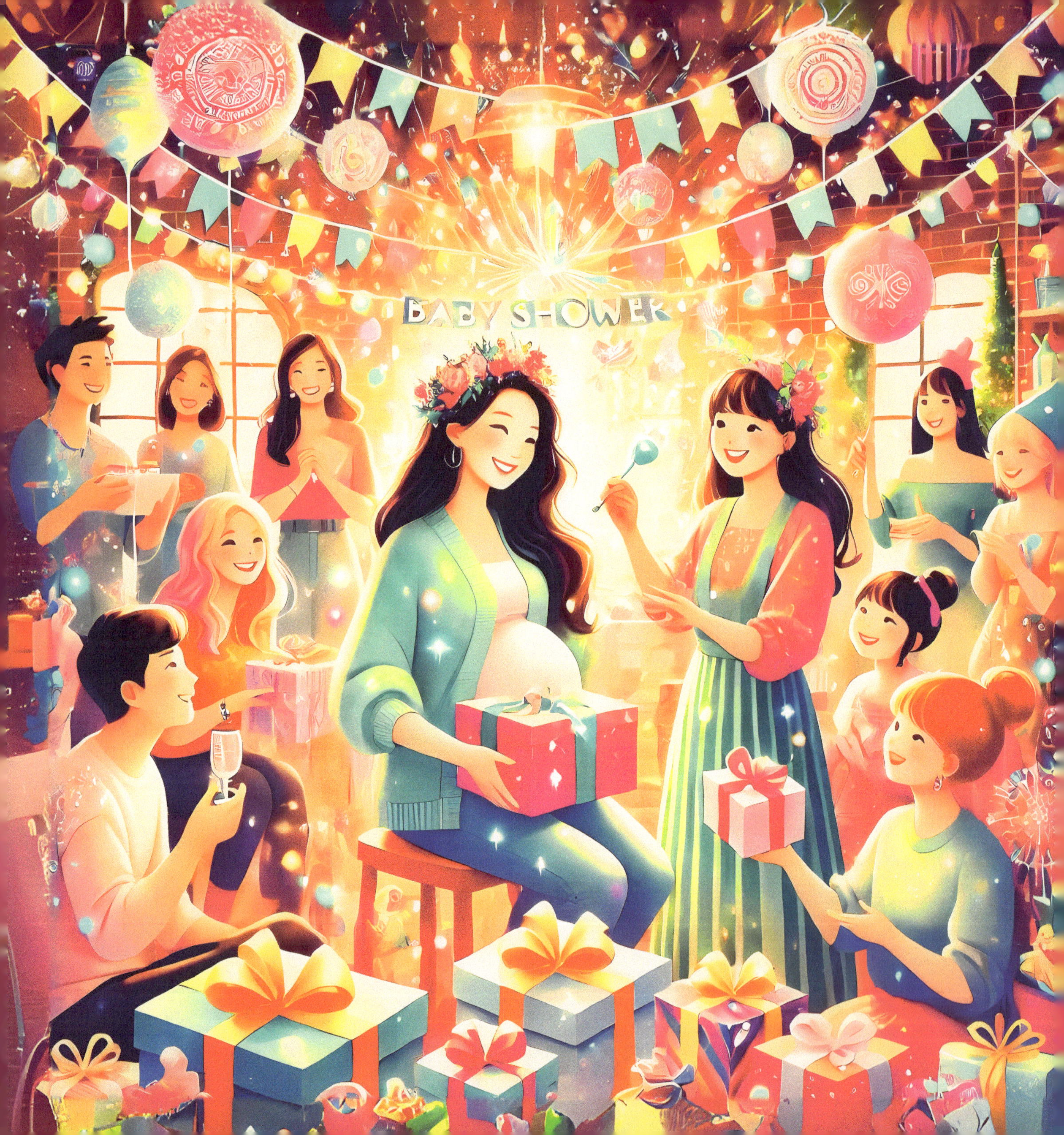

BABY SHOWER

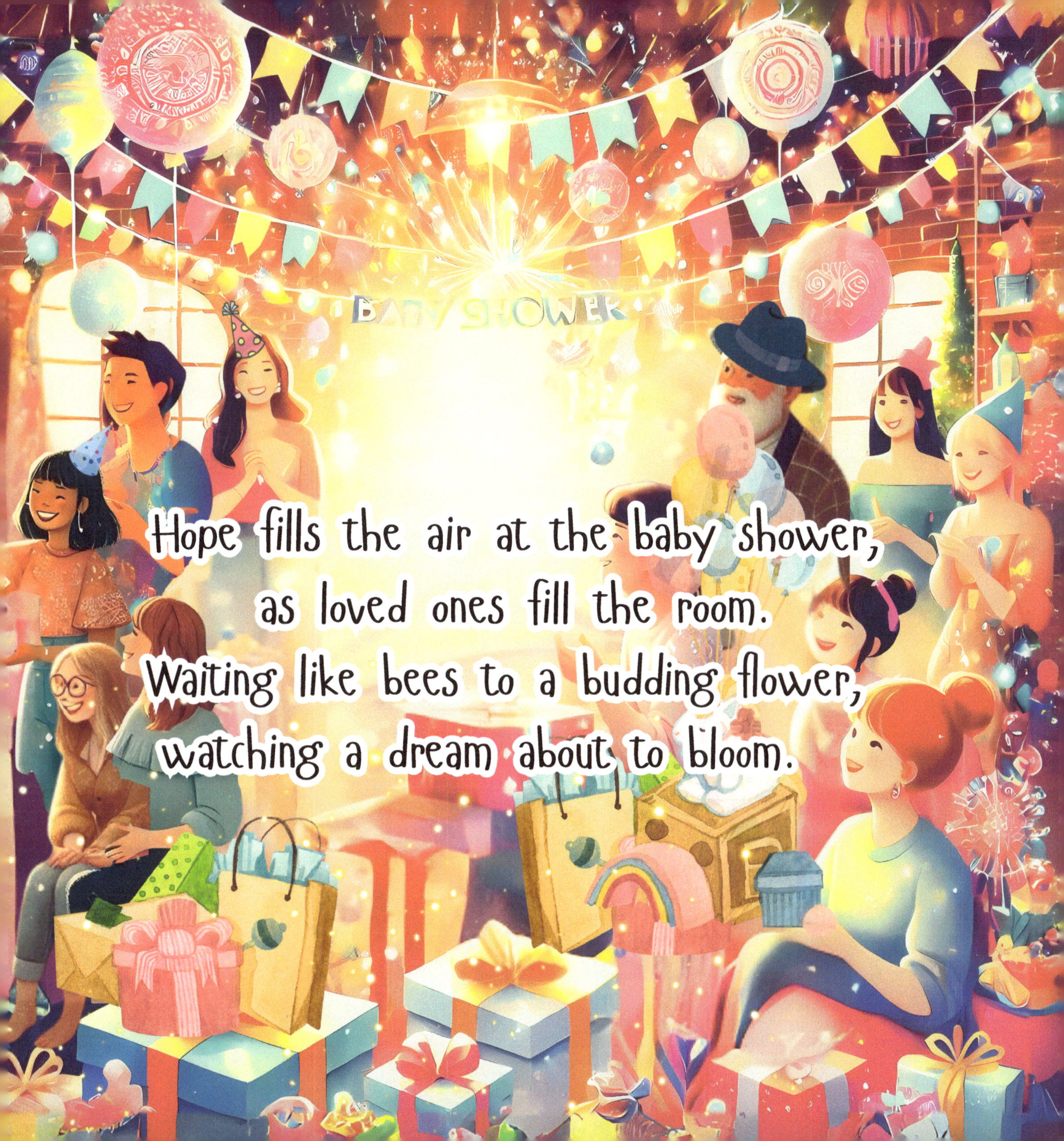

BABY SHOWER
Hope fills the air at the baby shower,
as loved ones fill the room.
Waiting like bees to a budding flower,
watching a dream about to bloom.

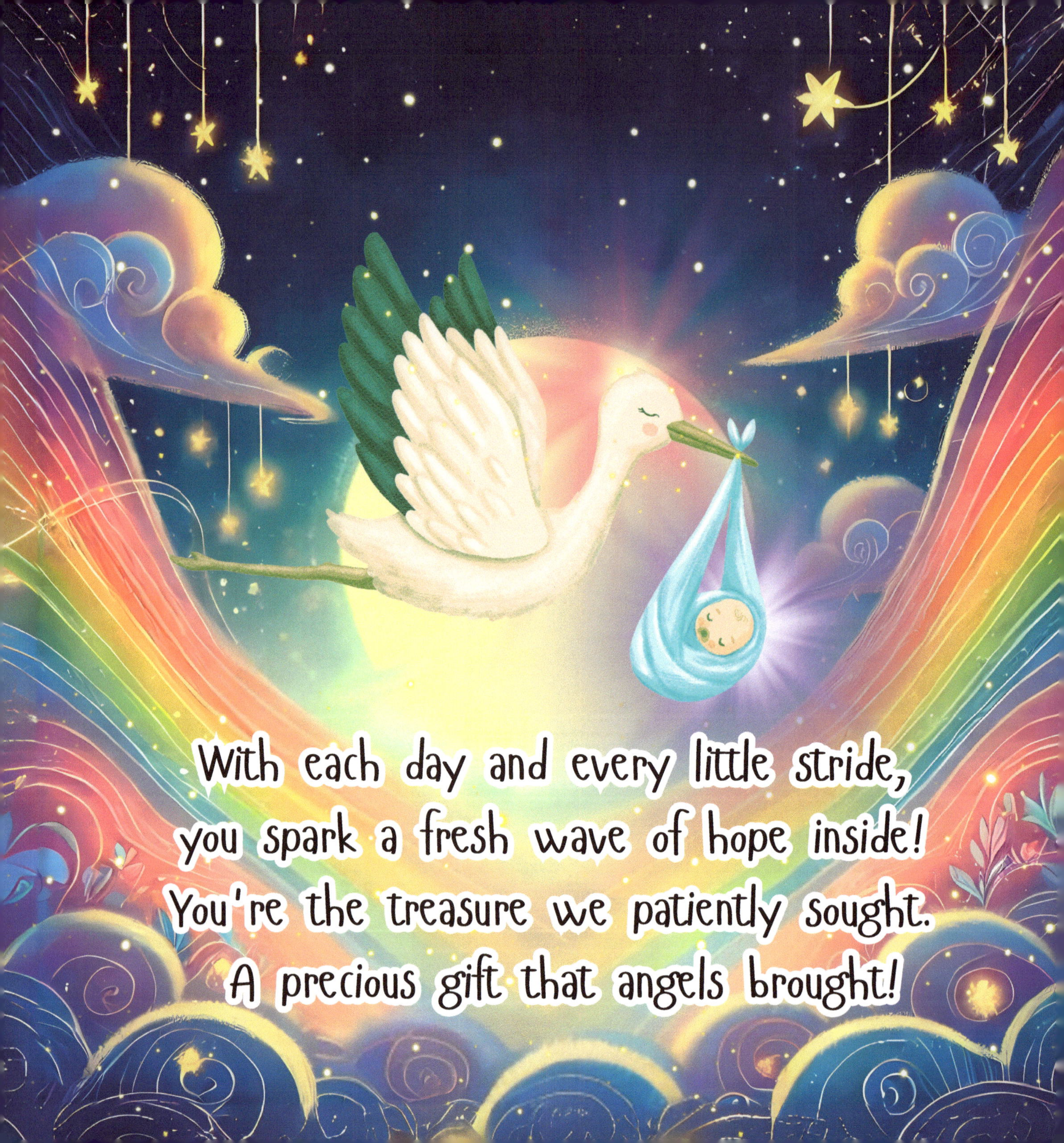

With each day and every little stride,
you spark a fresh wave of hope inside!
You're the treasure we patiently sought.
A precious gift that angels brought!

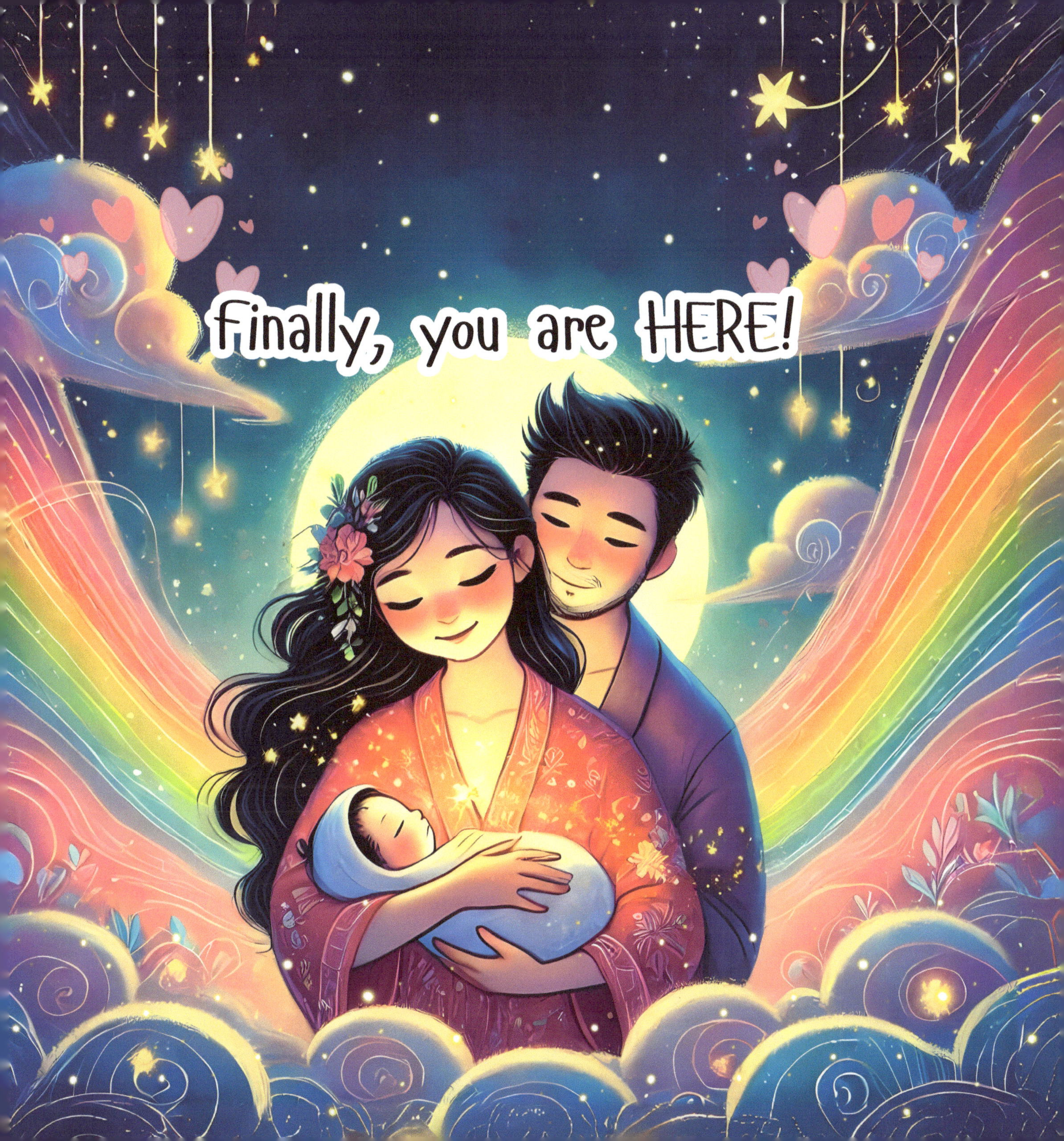
Finally, you are HERE!

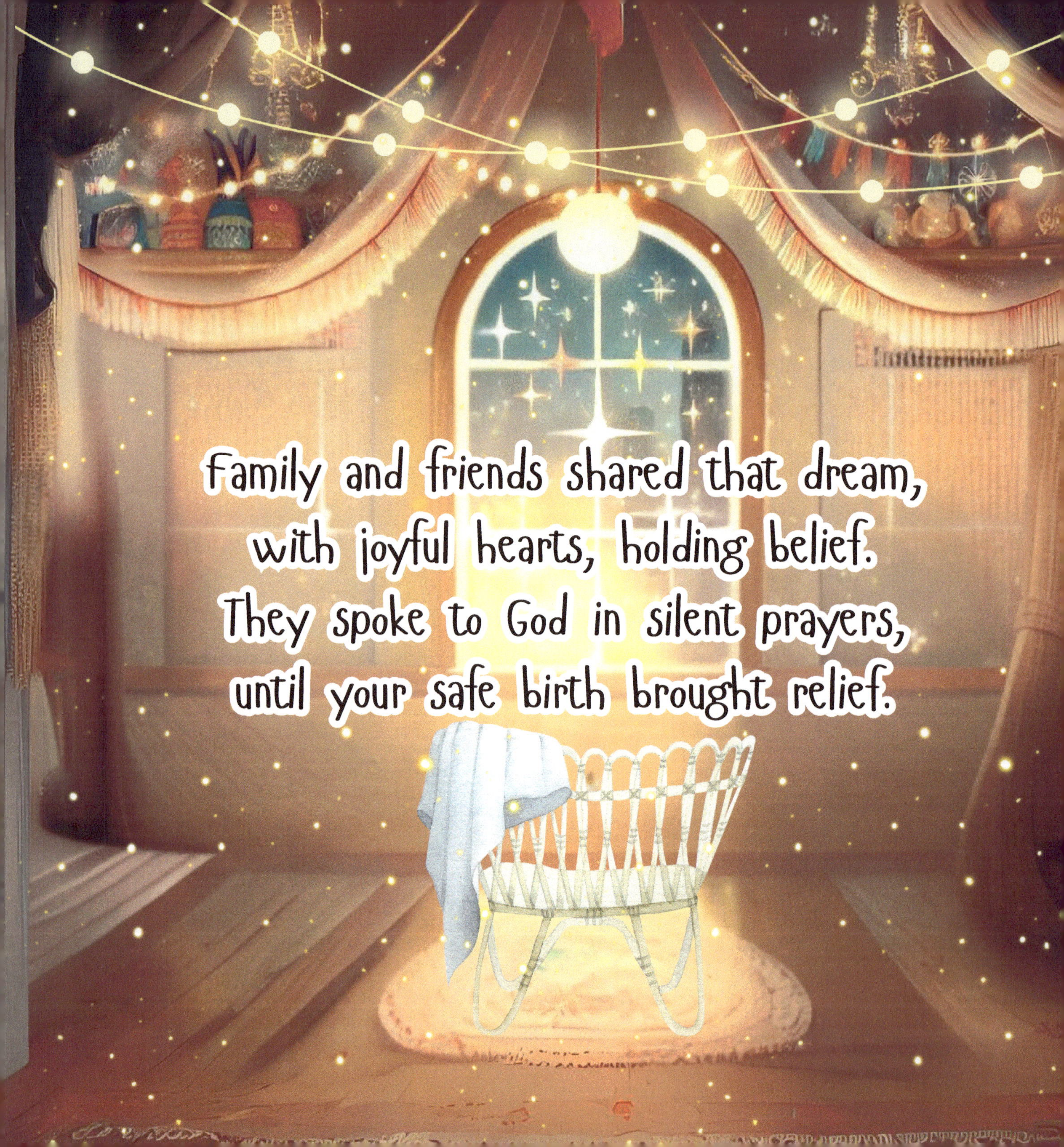

Family and friends shared that dream,
with joyful hearts, holding belief.
They spoke to God in silent prayers,
until your safe birth brought relief.

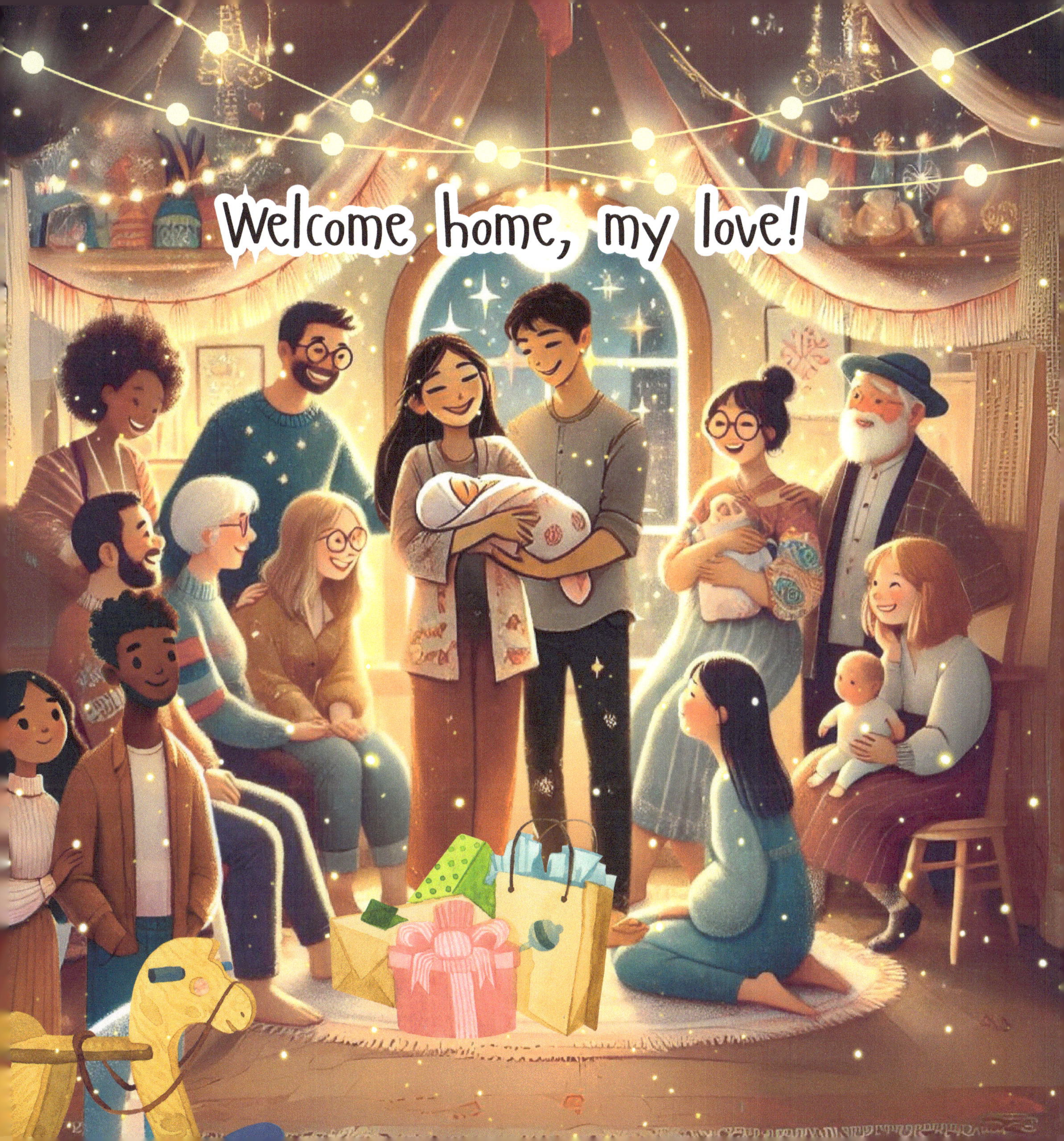

Welcome home, my love!

You fill our world with smiles,
not frowns.
Our love for you
knows no bounds.
It's deep as oceans, so vast and true,

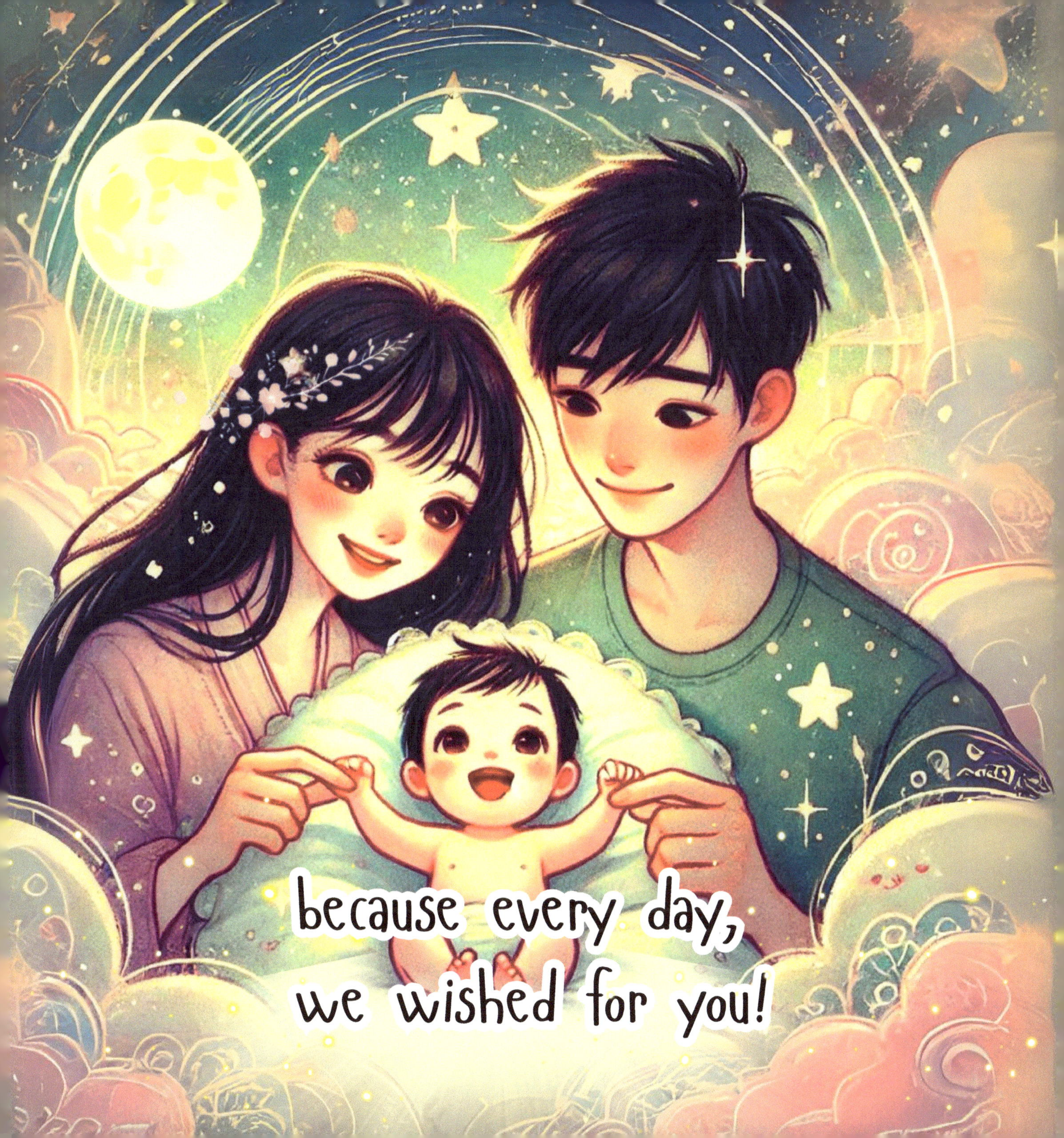
because every day,
we wished for you!

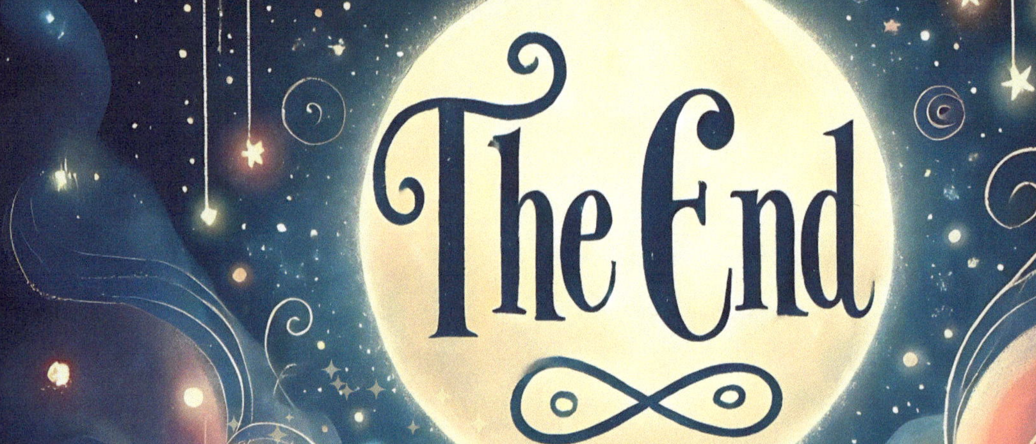
The End

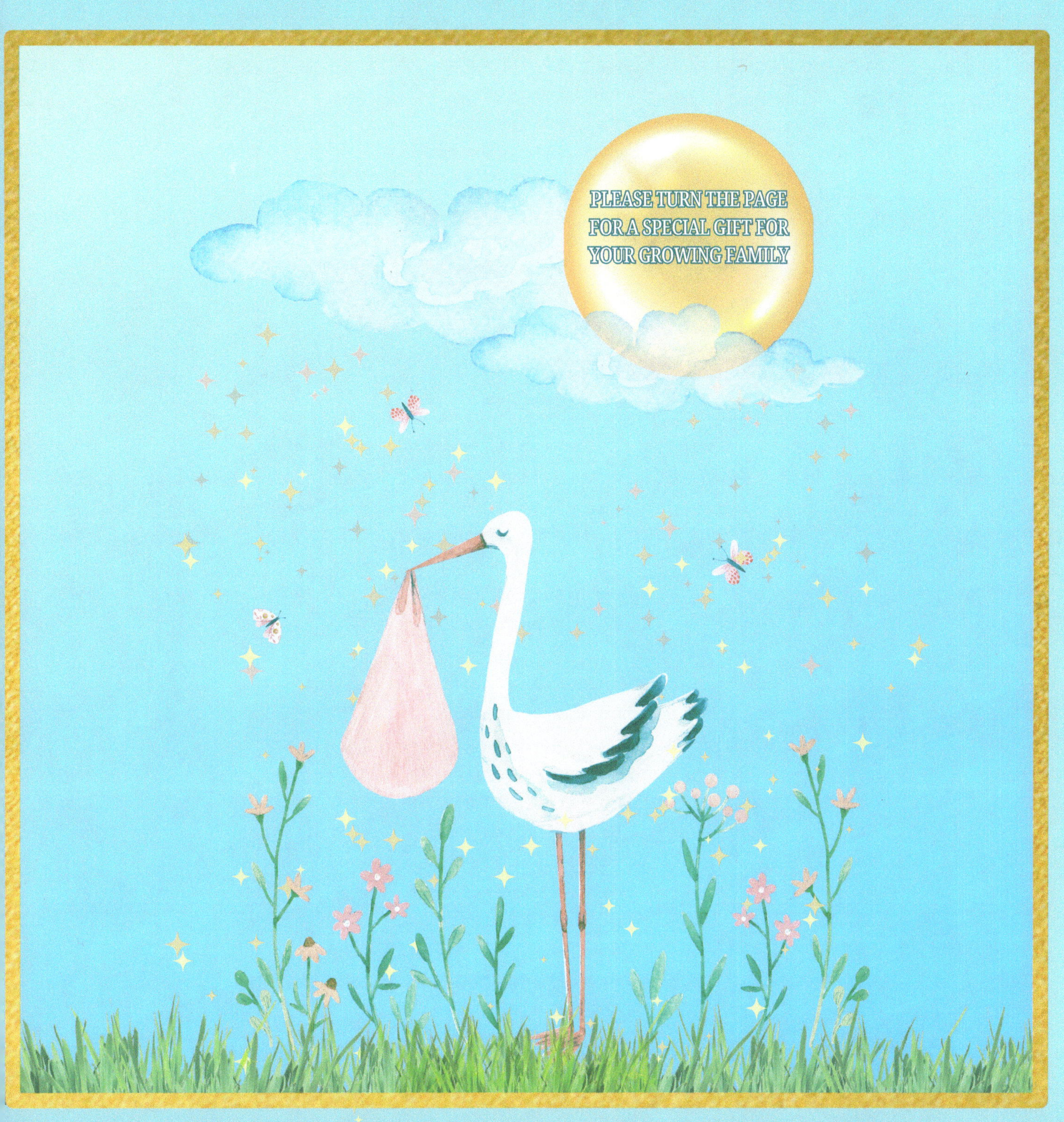
PLEASE TURN THE PAGE
FOR A SPECIAL GIFT FOR
YOUR GROWING FAMILY

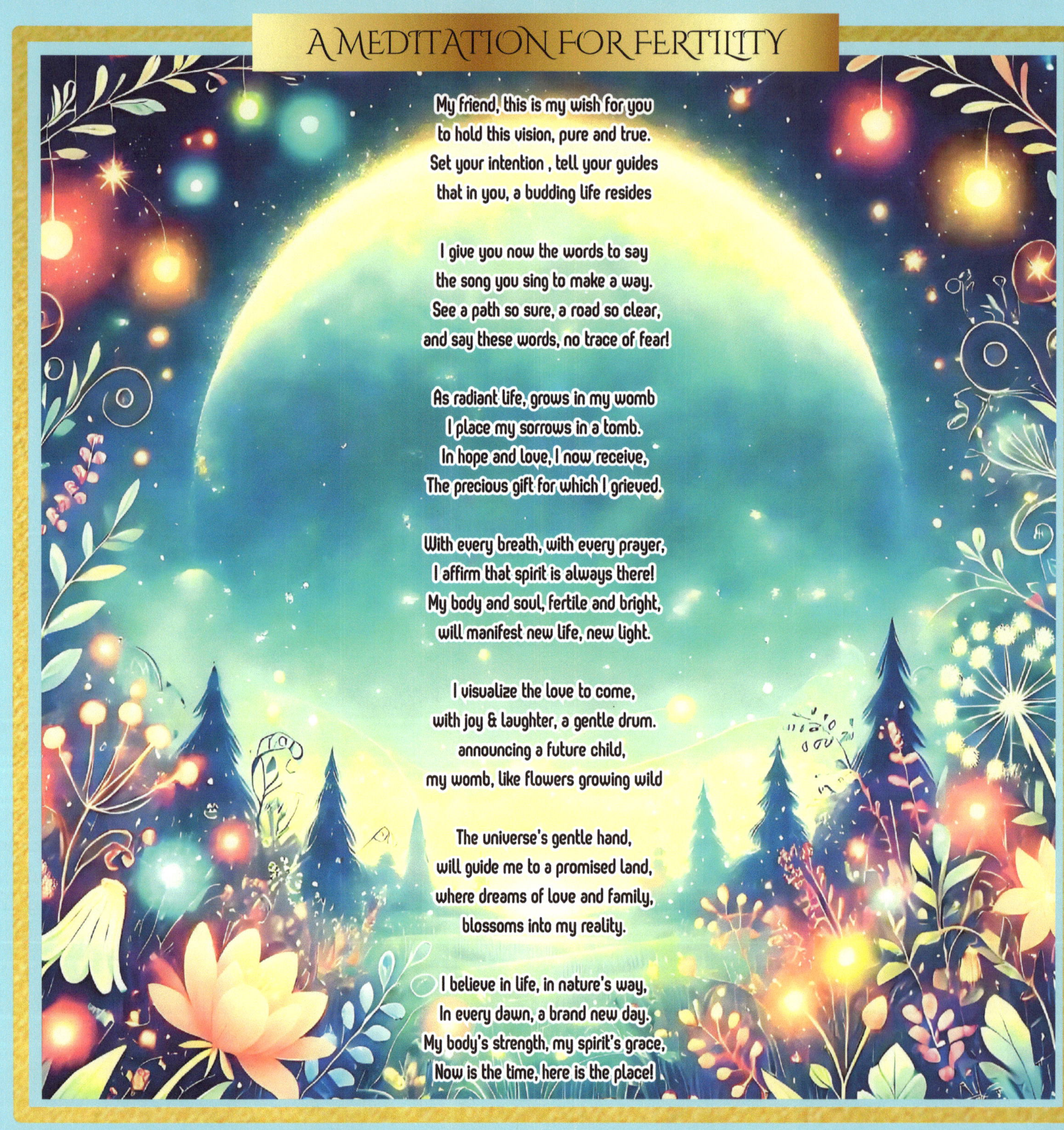

A MEDITATION FOR FERTILITY

My friend, this is my wish for you
to hold this vision, pure and true.
Set your intention , tell your guides
that in you, a budding life resides

I give you now the words to say
the song you sing to make a way.
See a path so sure, a road so clear,
and say these words, no trace of fear!

As radiant life, grows in my womb
I place my sorrows in a tomb.
In hope and love, I now receive,
The precious gift for which I grieved.

With every breath, with every prayer,
I affirm that spirit is always there!
My body and soul, fertile and bright,
will manifest new life, new light.

I visualize the love to come,
with joy & laughter, a gentle drum.
announcing a future child,
my womb, like flowers growing wild

The universe's gentle hand,
will guide me to a promised land,
where dreams of love and family,
blossoms into my reality.

I believe in life, in nature's way,
In every dawn, a brand new day.
My body's strength, my spirit's grace,
Now is the time, here is the place!

- This meditation is designed to help you release thoughts and energies that may weigh you down, particularly during times when your desire to become a parent feels most intense. As you read the verses, your vibrations will elevate you to envision and feel your body having everything it needs to support a healthy pregnancy and beyond.

- Begin this meditation by finding a quiet, comfortable spot to sit.

- Take several slow, deep breaths (inhale for 4 seconds, exhale for 5 seconds). Continue this cycle as long as needed to achieve relaxation.

- Once you feel relaxed, start reading the meditation quietly to yourself or aloud.

- As you read, try to visualize the imagery that the affirmations convey. Picture it happening for you in your mind's eye, and feel the emotions associated with each scene. Savor the sensation of receiving what you are manifesting, and express gratitude to the universe in your heart and mind.

- Feel free to repeat this meditation as often as you wish, especially during moments of doubt.

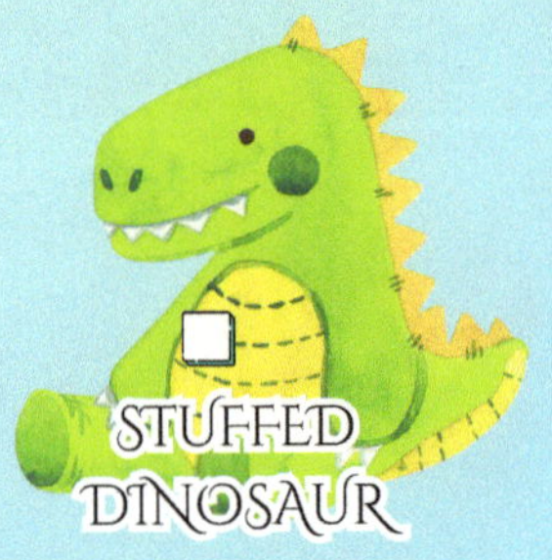

STUFFED DINOSAUR

BLUE PAINT

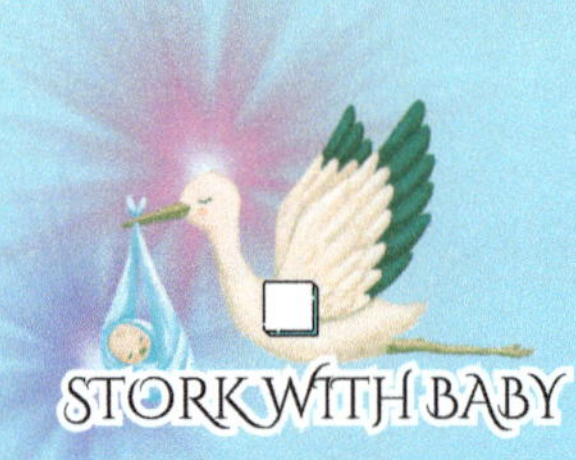

STORK WITH BABY

FULL MOON

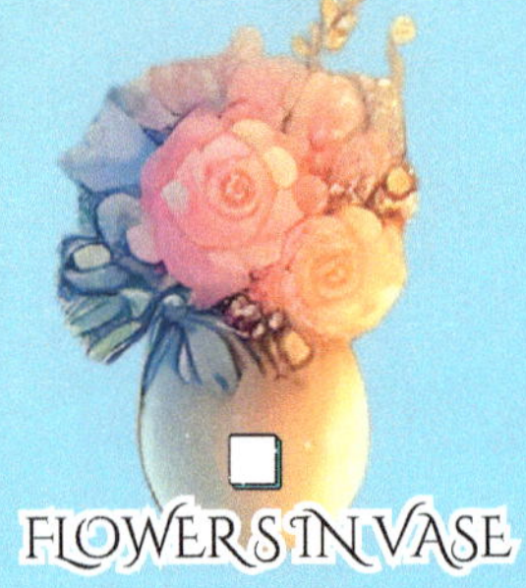

FLOWERS IN VASE

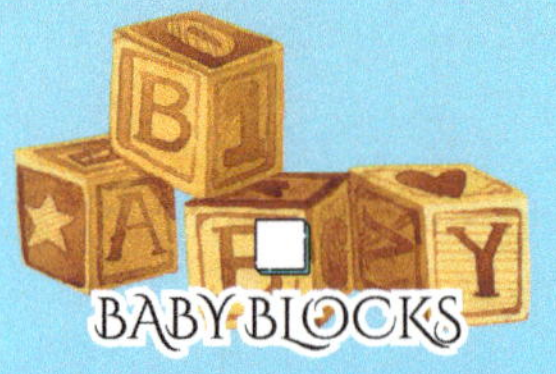

BABY BLOCKS

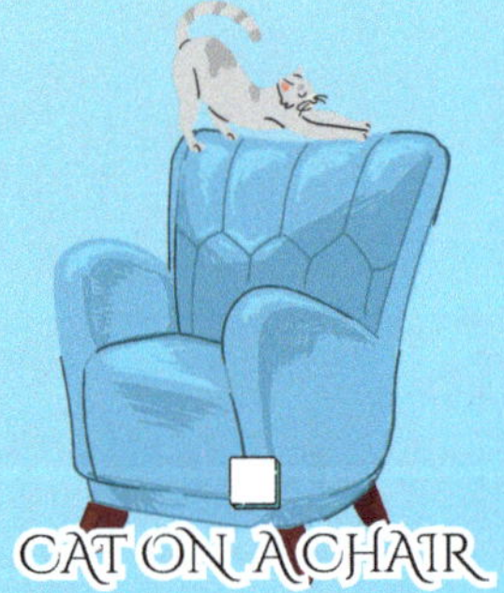

CAT ON A CHAIR

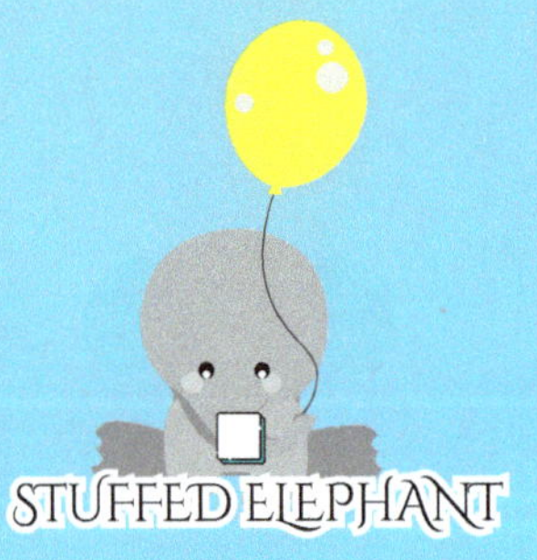

STUFFED ELEPHANT

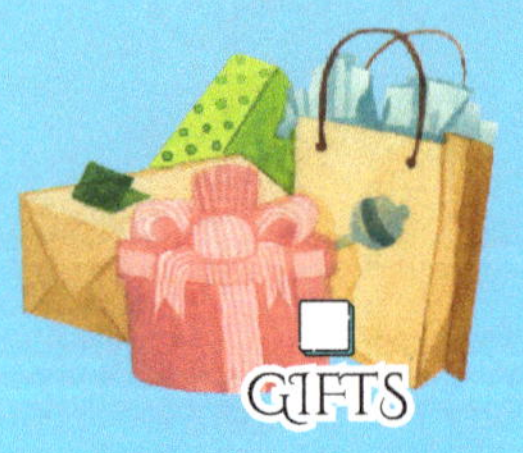

GIFTS

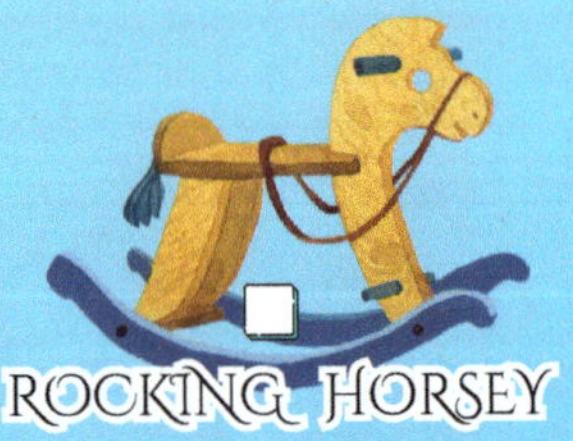

ROCKING HORSEY

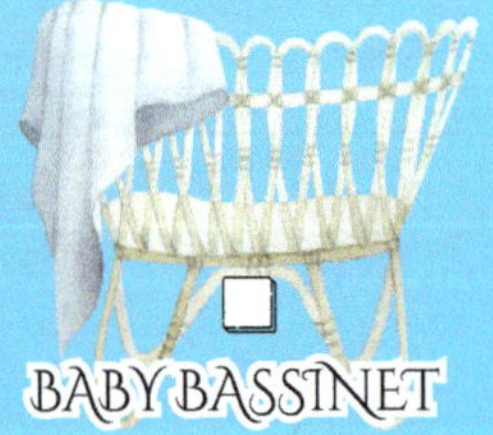

BABY BASSINET

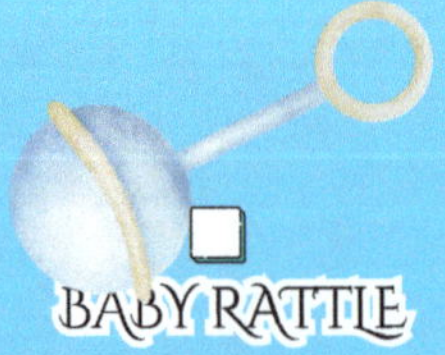

BABY RATTLE

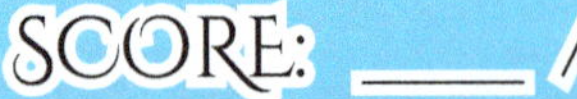

SCORE: _____ /12

Hi, friend!
My name is Christina. I 'm a nurse and intuitive development coach. I love art and writing, so I create journals, self-love workbooks, guided meditations, and workshops. Each book is designed with the intention to infuse a little joy, spark some gratitude, and sow seeds of love into your day! I want to keep in touch. Visit my author page on Amazon, or message me on social media:

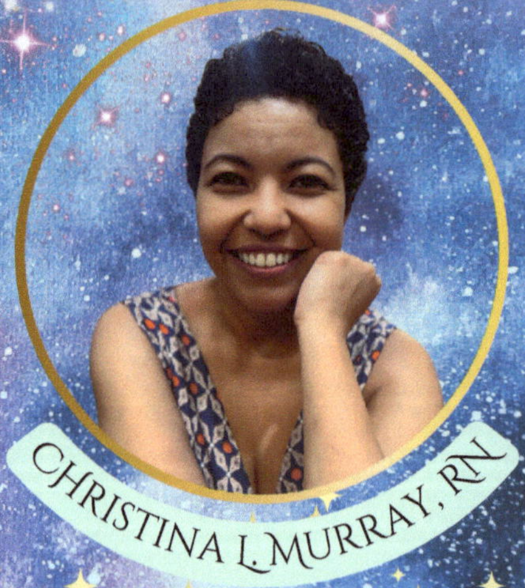

https://www.amazon.com/author/clmurraybooks

Channel: Infin8RN

@Infin8RN

OpenHeartsandSafeSpaces on Tiktok